# Packed Lunches & Snacks

The British Diabetic Association's Home Economist provides a wealth of delicious recipes ranging from day-to-day packed meals for school and work to elaborate picnics.

*By the same author*
THE DIABETIC'S MICROWAVE COOKBOOK

# Packed Lunches & Snacks

## Delicious Recipes for the Diabetic's Lunch Box

### Sue Hall

*Illustrated by Ian Jones*

THORSONS PUBLISHING GROUP
Wellingborough, Northamptonshire
—————— · ——————
Rochester, Vermont

BRITISH DIABETIC ASSOCIATION
London

First published June 1986
Second Impression August 1986

The British Library Cataloguing in Publication Data

Hall, Sue
    Packed lunches and snacks: delicious recipes
    for the diabetic's lunch box.
    1. Diabetics — Diet therapy — Recipes
    2. Lunchbox cookery
    I. Title    II. British Diabetic Association
    641.5'6314    RC662

    ISBN 0-7225-1283-X

Printed and bound in Great Britain

# Acknowledgements

The British Diabetic Association would like to acknowledge the generosity of G. D. Searle & Co. Ltd and Vitalia Ltd in supplying samples of their sweeteners for recipe testing, and Miss Claire Turner for her help with recipe development.

# Contents

## Recipes

Throughout the book I have used this standard conversion chart:

### Weights

25g — 1 oz
50g — 2 oz
75g — 3 oz
100g — 4 oz
150g — 5 oz
175g — 6 oz
200g — 7 oz
225g — 8 oz
250g — 9 oz
275g — 10 oz
300g — 11 oz
350g — 12 oz
375g — 13 oz
400g — 14 oz
425g — 15 oz
450g — 16 oz

### Liquid Measures

150ml — ¼ pint
275ml — ½ pint
425ml — ¾ pint
550ml — 1 pint

### Spoon Measures

1 teaspoon — 5ml
1 tablespoon — 15ml

It is best to use this to get accurate results.

Comparative Oven Temperatures are given below:

### Oven Temperatures

| Fahrenheit | Centigrade | Gas |
| --- | --- | --- |
| 300° | 150° | No 2 |
| 325° | 160° | No 3 |
| 350° | 180° | No 4 |
| 375° | 190° | No 5 |
| 400° | 200° | No 6 |
| 425° | 220° | No 7 |
| 450° | 230° | No 8 |

# Introduction

Fitting diabetes into normal life is everyone's goal, but it is all too easy for the routine meals to become monotonous. Snacks can be a particular problem. After living with a diabetic teenager and helping at many BDA Camps with a wide range of children, I can see why people often find snacks boring and difficult. It is easy to slip into the habit of making bad food choices at snack time. Bags and bags of crisps and lots of chocolate biscuits may seem easy to carry and eat but they really don't fit well into our dietary aims of high fibre and low fat. The odd bag of crisps is not impossible to justify but there are lots of 'healthier' alternatives and better food choices — many of which I found worked well with teenagers and children alike.

If, at the moment, your packed lunches and snacks look like this:

Sausage roll
Cheese in white bread sandwiches
Crisps
Chocolate biscuit
Can of drink

Why not make a few subtle changes to:

Wholemeal sausage roll
Reduced fat cheese in granary bread sandwiches
Wholewheat crisps or fruit and cereal snack bar
Home-baked high-fibre cake or biscuit
Sugar-free carbonated drink

By making a few substitutions you have increased the fibre and decreased the fat in your packed lunch. Altogether more healthy!

The aim of this book then, is to provide a selection of recipes and ideas to liven up 'packing and snacking' and to help us keep to a reduced fat/higher fibre diet while counting carbohydrate and/or calories — and enjoying ourselves!

To ensure good control of diabetes we need to eat regularly and in the correct quantities. Most of you will have a prescribed carbohydrate and/or calorie allowance and you *must* stick to this. Also if you are advised to have snacks in between meals you should have them. They help to keep you 'balanced!' — and good balance is very important.

*Remember* you are aiming for a high-fibre, low-fat, low-sugar diet within your dietary allowances, so *all* of your food choices are important.

## Why is Fibre so Important in our Food Choices?

You will see many references in current advice to diabetics about fibre in the diet. There is a lot of evidence to suggest that a diet with a good proportion of its carbohydrate coming from fibre-rich carbohydrate is really helpful in controlling blood sugar levels — helping to prevent low or high blood sugars and generally improving control. Diabetics who follow a high-fibre diet do seem to find their control improves and the decrease in 'hypos' is welcomed by everyone. Also, of course, it is generally healthier to eat plenty of fibre-rich foods. The recipes and advice here then is aimed at helping you to improve the quality of your carbohydrate intake.

## What About Fat?

It is now generally accepted that most of us would benefit from eating less fat and in having vegetable rather than animal fats. A fairly low total fat intake is therefore part of a good eating plan for all of us. Our recipes will help you to lower your total fat intake.

## The Recipes

All the recipes show the total carbohydrate and calorie content and a suggestion of number of portions. A freezing note is added to help planning. All the recipes are thoroughly tested. All spoon measures are level and you should only use the *Imperial* or the *Metric* measurements — not mix the two (the recipes have been calculated on the Imperial measurements). Some of the recipes use ingredients you may not have used before so the details below may be helpful.

*Flour*
(a) Wholemeal and Wholemeal Self-Raising. These are 100% wholemeal flour — they contain lots of fibre and are very useful for pastry, bread and cakes. The self-raising version should always be used if it is specified in a recipe.

(b) 81% Plain and Self-Raising. The figure 81 per cent refers to the extraction rates of the flour during milling, i.e. the amount of the grain left in the flour. These, therefore, contain less fibre than wholemeal but more than white flour. They are a good compromise choice and often produce lighter results than wholemeal. If a recipe specifies 81% then this should be used. These flours are made by several companies and are available in health food stores and many supermarkets.

*Low-Fat Spread/Margarine*
Always try to use a low-fat spread of vegetable origin — e.g. sunflower low-fat spread. These are now widely available in many supermarkets. Some recipes mention margarine, not a low-fat spread. If this is specified it should always be used because the recipe requires it.

*Fructose (Fruit Sugar)*
This is a bulk sweetener sold under the brand names of *Dietade* or *Fructofin* in chemists and supermarkets. In our recipes we have followed normal BDA policy of not counting the carbohydrate so long as one does not have more than 1 oz (25g) per day. If you use lots of our recipes in one day you will need to bear in mind the amount of fructose you are eating. The calories in fructose are always counted.

**Hints for Packed Lunches**
There is no reason why a meal or a snack away from home need be

any less appetizing than one eaten at home. Several basic rules for packing can help to keep food in tip top condition.

1.  Choose your containers carefully. Several firms now produce specifically designed plastic boxes in many shapes and sizes which are, of course, really useful. However, empty ice cream or margarine boxes are also well worth saving. Plastic sandwich bags however should only ever be used once — never washed.

2.  Wrap foods such as bread or cake tightly in film wrap to keep them moist and fresh. I have designed the recipes to be fairly sturdy but try to position things so foods won't get too crushed.

3.  For a freeze-ahead lunch choose a range of foods which all freeze well, pack them up and freeze the whole box — remember to allow adequate time for thawing.

4.  Apply the same rules about a variety of colours and textures as you would to a meal at home. I find lots of colourful items such as vegetables and fruit add interest to a lunch box.

5.  Follow the guidelines in Chapter 1 to intermingle 'bought' and everyday foods to get the best from both.

6.  Try not to get stuck in a rut by always selecting the same foods — use the recipes to really ring the changes.

# 1. Balancing Packed Meals

As well as ensuring your meal or snack contains the correct amount of carbohydrate and/or the right number of calories, it is important to use a variety of foods to ensure you eat enough fibre and not too much fat. The recipes I have developed are all fairly high in fibre and as low in fat as I can make them so they are ideal for planning healthy meals for the whole family. However, it is also important to be able to use a mixture of bought and home-made foods, so I have given you some advice on that too.

The following lists give some ideas for using a range of everyday foods and 'bought' foods in packed meals.

## Using Everyday Foods

**(a) Bread and Bread Products** — try to use wholemeal/granary. Always a good basis for a packed meal and snack. The individual products have different carbohydrate (CHO) and calorie (Cals) values, many of which are given on the packaging, but as a general guide:

*Uncut Bread:*
1 oz (25g) wholemeal bread contains 10g CHO and 50 calories
1 oz (25g) white       bread contains 15g CHO and 65 calories

*Sliced Bread:*
If your sliced bread doesn't have a CHO and calorie count on the packet you can assume:

| | Wholemeal/ Granary | | White | |
|---|---|---|---|---|
| | CHO | Cals | CHO | Cals |
| 1 large thick slice | 19g | 90 | 20g | 100 |
| 1 large medium slice | 15g | 70 | 15g | 75 |
| 1 large thin slice | N/A | N/A | 14g | 65 |
| 1 small slice | 10g | 55 | 14g | 65 |
| 1 roll | 20g | 130 | 30g | 140 |

1 average wholemeal pitta bread contains 40g CHO and 180 calories.
1 average white    pitta bread contains 40g CHO and 230 calories.

**(b) Dairy Products** — a major source of fat in the diet. Care has to be taken here to avoid too much fat. The following products are fairly low in fat.

| | Quantity | CHO | Cals |
|---|---|---|---|
| Cottage cheese | 1 oz (25g) | neg | 25 |
| Reduced fat cottage cheese | 1 oz (25g) | neg | 25 |
| Reduced fat hard cheese | 1 oz (25g) | neg | 70 |
| Reduced fat soft cheese | 1 oz (25g) | neg | 40 |
| Curd cheese | 1 oz (25g) | neg | 40 |
| Quark cheese | 1 oz (25g) | 1½g | 55 |
| Milk | 1 pint (550ml) | 30g | 370 |
| Milk (semi skimmed) | 1 pint (550ml) | 30g | 260 |
| Milk (skimmed) | 1 pint (550ml) | 30g | 190 |
| Low fat milk | 1 pint (550ml) | 30g | 250 |
| Soya drink (sugar free) | 500ml carton | neg | 185 |
| Natural low-fat yogurt | 5 oz (150g) pot | 10g | 80 |
| Typical 'diet' yogurt | 5 oz (150g) pot | av 10g (8-13g) | 85 |
| Sweetened fruit yogurt | 5 oz (150g) pot | variable | |
| Low fat spreads | 1 oz (25g) | neg | 100 |
| Margarines | 1 oz (25g) | neg | 180 |
| Butter | 1 oz (25g) | neg | 185 |

(Always try to use a low-fat spread.)

## (c) **Eggs**

Very packable by themselves and useful for fillings etc.

|  | CHO | Cals |
|---|---|---|
| Egg (1×Size 2) | *neg* | 80 |

## (d) **Fruit**

There is a large range of fresh and dried fruits available, many of which are really useful in packed meals and snacks. A few are listed below — *all giving 10g CHO.*

|  | Quantity | CHO | Cals |
|---|---|---|---|
| Apple — eating | 1 medium | 10g | 50 |
| Apricots — fresh | 3 medium | 10g | 40 |
| — dried | 4 small | 10g | 45 |
| Banana — peeled | 1 small | 10g | 40 |
| Cherries — fresh, whole | 12 | 10g | 40 |
| Currants — dried | ½ oz (12g) | 10g | 35 |
| Dates — fresh, whole | 3 medium | 10g | 40 |
| — dried, stoned | 3 small | 10g | 40 |
| Grapes | 10 large | 10g | 40 |
| Guavas | 1 | 10g | 45 |
| Mango | ⅓ of large | 10g | 40 |
| Melon | large slice | 10g | 40 |
| Nectarine | 1 | 10g | 40 |
| Oranges | 1 | 10g | 40 |
| Peach — fresh | 1 | 10g | 40 |
| Pear — fresh | 1 large | 10g | 40 |
| Plums — fresh | 2 large | 10g | 40 |
| Prunes — dried, stoned | 2 large | 10g | 40 |
| Raisins — dried | ½ oz (12g) | 10g | 35 |
| Raspberries | 6 oz (175g) | 10g | 45 |
| Strawberries — fresh | 5 oz (150g) (about 15) | 10g | 40 |
| Sultanas — dried | ½ oz (12g) | 10g | 40 |
| Tangerines — fresh | 2 large | 10g | 40 |

Ring the changes with a few of the more unusual fruits.

## (e) Fruit Juices

These are useful drinks but they do contain calories and the carbohydrate in them is quickly absorbed. They therefore need to be used with food as part of a snack or meal — not instead of one. It is best to drink fruit juices at the end of a meal or snack rather than at the beginning. Always choose an *unsweetened* fruit juice.

|                  | *Quantity*    | *CHO* | *Cals* |
|------------------|---------------|-------|--------|
| Apple juice      | 200ml carton  | 25g   | 90     |
| Grapefruit juice | 200ml carton  | 20g   | 80     |
| Orange juice     | 200ml carton  | 20g   | 80     |
| Pineapple juice  | 200ml carton  | 25g   | 90     |

## (f) Vegetables

Fresh, raw vegetables are always a good idea to include — just wash them well and peel only when absolutely necessary. Some of the most 'packable' contain so little carbohydrate and so few calories they need not be counted if a normal helping is eaten, for example, beansprouts, cabbage, carrots, celery, cucumber, lettuce, mushrooms, peppers, radishes, spring onions, tomatoes.

## (g) Using 'Bought' Foods

If you choose carefully then there is no reason why many convenience foods cannot be part of a healthy diet, but it can be difficult without knowing their carbohydrate and calorie content. The BDA's book *Countdown* (see Suggested Reading List) gives the figures for over 5000 foods. It uses the 'traffic light system':

*Think of your diet instructions as a set of traffic lights directing your diet:*
GREEN *for foods you should use;*
AMBER *for foods you can use with caution;*
RED *(for foods which shouldn't be used regularly but may be used on special occasions).*

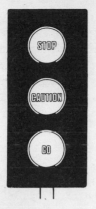

RED — STOP
Don't use these foods except on special occasions.

AMBER — CAUTION
Use these foods with care and not as the largest part of the diet.

GREEN — GO
Use these foods regularly.

The following are all Green 'GO' versions of foods (i.e. low in fat and sugar, high in fibre) and useful to include.

Biscuits — try to choose those using wholemeal flour and as little sugar as possible. See the ingredient list on the pack and the Green Section of *Countdown*.

Cakes and Teabreads — not as inexpensive as making your own, but many firms now produce wholemeal cakes and teabreads. Examples of a 'typical' product are given below:

|  | CHO | Calories |
|---|---|---|
| Wholemeal fruited muffins (1) | 30- 35g | 140-160 |
| Wholemeal fruited scones (1) | 25- 30g | 160-200 |
| Wholemeal fruited teabuns (1) | 30g | 170 |
| Wholemeal fruited teacakes (1) | 30g | 160-170 |
| Wholemeal malt loaf (1) | 125-135g | 570-580 |
| Wholemeal plain scone (1) | 20- 25g | 150-170 |

Drinks — low calorie squash and carbonated drinks are very useful for packing up and extremely suitable.

Canned Fish — a good standby for fillings etc. — always look for products in brine — *not* oil — to help keep the fat content down.

**Canned Fruit** — fruit in water or natural juice are useful as bases for jellies or in fruit salads. Always look for *natural juice* rather than syrup.

**Salads** — if you don't want to make your own salads there are several available which are suitable for packing and as part of your diet — look in the Green Section of *Countdown*.

**Snack Bars** — these are often a convenient way to carry a snack or part of a lunch, there are a wide range available, some of which are more suitable than others! Look on the ingredients list and avoid those with too much added sugar — this could be in the form of sucrose, honey or fruit juice, and if the content is high these sugars will appear near the beginning of the list. Their values range between 10-25g CHO and 75-150 calories. It is important, therefore, to check the figures on the pack or in the BDA's book *Countdown*. Also look out for high-fibre alternatives to crisps.

Also useful are products like ready-prepared wholemeal pizza bases, pure fruit spreads, low-sugar/reduced sugar jams and peanut butter.

# 2. Bread and Bread Products

*Lots of healthy home-made goods to try — with over twenty new fillings for your lunches and snacks*

## Bread Packets

---

Makes 15 packets    Total CHO — 240g    Total Cals — 1200

---

½ oz (12g) low-fat spread
¾ lb (350g) 81% flour
1 teaspoon sea salt
½ sachet 'quick acting yeast'
8 fl oz (220ml) hand hot water

**1.** Rub fat into flour, add salt and yeast. Stir in hand hot water and knead for 10 minutes. Cut into 15.

**2.** Roll bread out flat on lightly oiled trays, cover and leave to rise for 1 hour.

**3.** Using one of the five fillings given on pages 20-23, place 2 tablespoons of filling onto each base, brush the edges of the base with water and fold up.

**4.** Bake at 425°F/220°C (Gas Mark 7) for 15 minutes or until brown. Allow to cool on a wire rack.

Each bread packet contains 15g CHO and 80 calories — *remember* to add the filling figures to this, depending on your choice of filling.

*Note:* This recipe freezes well.

The following fillings are also suitable for use in rolls, sandwiches, pittas and Pancake Parcels (see page 43). Remember to add their carbohydrate and calorie figures to your base.

# Chicken and Sweetcorn Filling

Fills 15 packets     Total CHO — 60g     Total Cals — 710

*1 oz (25g) low-fat spread*
*1 oz (25g) wholemeal flour*
*½ pint (275ml) skimmed milk*
*1 teaspoon thyme*
*8 oz (225g) cooked chicken, diced*
*8 oz (225g) sweetcorn*
*Sea salt and freshly ground black pepper to taste*

**1.** Melt fat and add flour, cook for 2-3 minutes.
**2.** Slowly add milk to make a sauce.
**3.** Add the herbs, chicken and sweetcorn and combine thoroughly. Season to taste and use as required.

*Note:* This recipe freezes well.

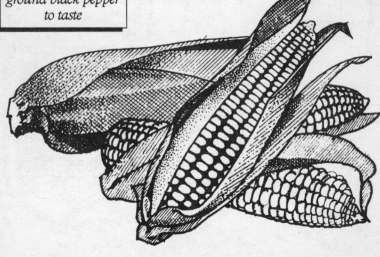

# Lentil Curry Filling

| Fills 15 packets | Total CHO — 60g | Total Cals — 470 |
|---|---|---|

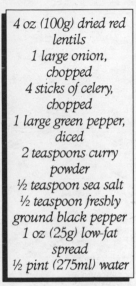

*4 oz (100g) dried red lentils*
*1 large onion, chopped*
*4 sticks of celery, chopped*
*1 large green pepper, diced*
*2 teaspoons curry powder*
*½ teaspoon sea salt*
*½ teaspoon freshly ground black pepper*
*1 oz (25g) low-fat spread*
*½ pint (275ml) water*

**1.** Boil the lentils in water in a semi-covered pan for 20 minutes until soft and quite thick — DO NOT allow to boil dry. Add more water if necessary.

**2.** Fry onion gently for 2-3 minutes, then add celery and green pepper and cook for a further 2-3 minutes.

**3.** Add cooked lentils and curry powder and stir thoroughly for 2 minutes. Use as required.

*Note:* This recipe freezes well.

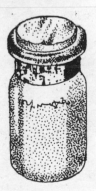

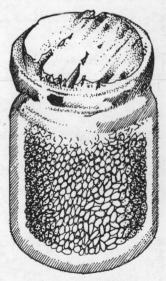

# Mushroom and Herb Filling ✓

Fills 15 packets     Total CHO — 10g     Total Cals — 200

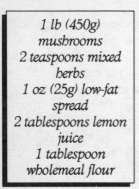

*1 lb (450g)
mushrooms
2 teaspoons mixed
herbs
1 oz (25g) low-fat
spread
2 tablespoons lemon
juice
1 tablespoon
wholemeal flour*

**1.** Sweat mushrooms with herbs in low-fat spread for 5 minutes in a covered pan.
**2.** Remove cover, add lemon juice and sprinkle on wholemeal flour, stirring continuously. Use as required.

*Note:* This recipe freezes well.

# Spinach and Sweetcorn Filling

Fills 15 packets     Total CHO — 55g     Total Cals — 430

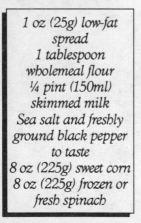

*1 oz (25g) low-fat
spread
1 tablespoon
wholemeal flour
¼ pint (150ml)
skimmed milk
Sea salt and freshly
ground black pepper
to taste
8 oz (225g) sweet corn
8 oz (225g) frozen or
fresh spinach*

**1.** Melt fat and stir in flour, and cook gently for 2-3 minutes.
**2.** Slowly stir in milk to make a sauce. Add salt, pepper, sweetcorn and spinach and combine thoroughly. Use as required.

*Note:* This recipe freezes well.

# Chilli Bean Filling ✓

---

Fills 15 packets     Total CHO — 40g     Total Cals — 290

---

½ oz (12g) low-fat spread
1 large onion, diced
1 red pepper, diced
2 tablespoons tomato purée
1 teaspoon chilli powder
8 oz (225g) red kidney beans — tinned

**1.** Sauté onion and red pepper for 2-3 minutes.
**2.** Add tomato purée and chilli powder. Add drained cooked red kidney beans and heat through. Use as required.

*Note:* This recipe freezes well.

# Sausage Bread Rolls          ✓

Makes 18          Total CHO — 185g          Total Cals — 1680

½ oz (12g) low-fat
spread
9 oz (250g) 81%
flour
¾ teaspoon sea salt
⅓ sachet 'fast acting
yeast'
5 fl oz (150ml) hand
hot water
8 oz (225g) good
quality sausage meat

**1.** Rub fat into flour, add salt and yeast, stir in water.

**2.** Knead for 10 minutes and allow to rise for 1 hour in a plastic bag.

**3.** Roll out sausage meat to one long sausage about ½ in (1cm) wide. (Use flour on your hands to stop sausagemeat sticking.)

**4.** Roll out bread to the same length as sausage meat and about three times as wide.

**5.** Place sausage meat in centre and fold edges. Seal and brush with skimmed milk.

**6.** Cut into 18 portions and place on a lightly oiled tray. Bake at 425°F/230°C (Gas Mark 7) for 15-20 minutes. Allow to cool on a wire rack.

Each sausage roll contains 10g CHO and 95 calories.

*Note:* This recipe freezes well.

# Mini Pizzas      ✓

---

Enough to top 8 roll halves  Total CHO — 40g  Total Cals — 480

---

### Base
4 medium wholemeal rolls — sliced horizontally

### Topping
1 large onion
½ oz (12g) low-fat spread
8 oz (225g) mushrooms
1 teaspoon mixed herbs
1×11 oz (300g) tin tomatoes, drained
1 tablespoon tomato purée
½ oz (12g) wholemeal flour
4 oz (100g) reduced-fat cheese, grated

**1.** Sauté the onion in the fat for 3-5 minutes until onion is soft.

**2.** Add mushrooms and herbs and gently cook for a further 5-10 minutes.

**3.** Add tomatoes and tomato purée and heat through thoroughly, breaking up the tomatoes.

**4.** Sprinkle on flour and thicken over a moderate heat for 3-5 minutes. Allow to cool slightly.

**5.** Cover the buns with topping and sprinkle with cheese. Grill for 2 minutes or bake at 350°F/180°C (Gas Mark 4) for 5 minutes. Allow to cool on a wire rack.

Add your share of the filling figures to the figures for your half of the roll.

*Note:* This recipe freezes well.

# Vegetarian Pizza

Makes 10 squares    Total CHO — 200g    Total Cals — 1180

**Base**
*9 oz (250g) 81%
flour
1 teaspoon sea salt
⅓ sachet 'fast acting
yeast'
½ oz (12g) low-fat
spread
5 fl oz (150ml) hand
hot water*

**1.** Mix flour, salt and yeast together, rub in fat. Add water and knead for 10 minutes. Roll out to line a baking tray, cover and leave to rise for 1 hour.

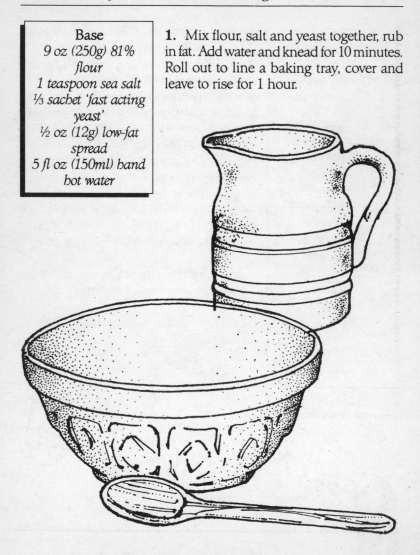

### Topping

1 large onion,
chopped
2 ~~cloves garlic~~,
crushed
1 oz (25g) low-fat
spread
1 teaspoon rosemary
1 teaspoon oregano
1 green pepper,
chopped
1 lb (450g)
mushrooms, sliced
1×12 oz (350g) tin
tomatoes
1 tablespoon tomato
purée
1 teaspoon wholemeal
flour
8 oz (225g) courgettes,
sliced
1 oz (25g) low-fat
spread
Sea salt and freshly
ground black pepper
to taste
5 oz (150g) tomatoes,
sliced

**2.** Fry onion and garlic in low-fat spread for 2-3 minutes. Add herbs, green pepper and mushrooms and fry for a further 5 minutes.

**3.** Add tinned tomatoes and purée and thicken with wholemeal flour. Leave to cool.

**4.** Chop courgettes and then fry in fat with some oregano, salt and pepper.

**5.** When base is risen, cover in mushroom mixture, top with courgettes and fresh tomatoes. Bake at 425°F/220°C (Gas Mark 7) for 20-25 minutes until base is crisp. Cut and allow to cool on a wire rack.

Each portion is 20g CHO and 120 calories.

*Note:* This recipe freezes well.

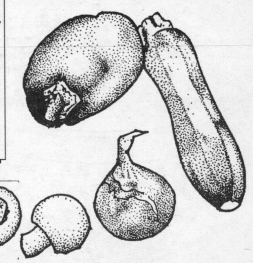

# Quick Brown Bread ✓

Makes 3×1 lb (450g) loaves *or* 34 small rolls
Total CHO — 510g          Total Cals — 2550

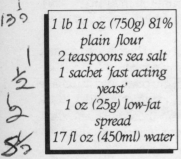

> 1 lb 11 oz (750g) 81%
> plain flour
> 2 teaspoons sea salt
> 1 sachet 'fast acting
> yeast'
> 1 oz (25g) low-fat
> spread
> 17 fl oz (450ml) water

**1.** Mix flour, salt and yeast. Rub in fat, add water and mix well. Knead for 10 minutes. Cover and leave to rise for 1 hour.

**For rolls:**
Shape into 34 equal size balls. Place on lightly oiled baking trays, cover and leave to rise until double in size. Bake at 375°F/190°C (Gas Mark 5) for 10-15 minutes. Allow to cool on a wire rack.

1 roll is 15g CHO and 75 calories.

**For loaves:**
Divide into 3 equal size pieces. Place each piece in a lightly oiled 1 lb (450g) loaf tin, cover and leave to rise until double in size. Bake at 375°F/190°C (Gas Mark 5) for 25-30 minutes until golden brown and hollow when tapped. Allow to cool on a wire rack.

Each loaf is 170g CHO and 850 calories.

*Note:* This recipe freezes well.

# Wholemeal Cheese and Bean Loaf

Slices into 8    Total CHO — 240g    Total Cals — 1600

2 oz (50g) low-fat spread
9 oz (250g) self-raising wholemeal flour
1 teaspoon mustard powder
1 teaspoon baking powder
1 teaspoon dried mixed herbs
3 oz (75g) reduced-fat hard cheese, grated
1×14 oz (400g) tin red brown (Borlotti) beans, drained
¼ pint (150ml) skimmed milk
1 size 3 egg

**1.** Rub fat into flour. Add mustard powder, baking powder and herbs. Stir in cheese and beans.

**2.** Beat milk and egg together, then mix thoroughly into mixture.

**3.** Turn into a lightly oiled and lined 2 lb (900g) loaf tin. Bake at 350°F/180°C (Gas Mark 4) for 45-60 minutes until firm. Allow to cool in the tin for 10 minutes. Turn out onto a wire rack.

Each slice is 30g CHO and 200 calories.

*Note:* This recipe freezes well.

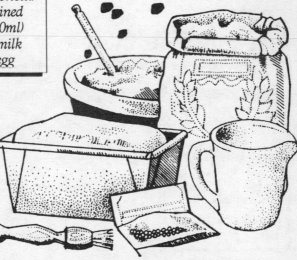

# Fillings

These fillings can all be used in rolls, sandwiches, pittas or pancakes. Remember to add their carbohydrate and calorie figures to your base.

## Tuna and Cucumber Filling ✓

Fills 4 large rolls or 3 pittas
Total CHO — *negligible*          Total Cals — 280

| | |
|---|---|
| 1×8 oz (227g) tin of tuna in brine, drained 1 oz (25g) low-fat spread ¼ cucumber, diced | Flake tuna, blend with low-fat spread, add diced cucumber. Chill and use as required. Any excess mixture could be stored for up to 2 days covered in a refrigerator. *Note:* This recipe is *not* suitable for freezing. |

## Egg and Ham Filling ✓

Fills 3 large rolls or 2 pittas
Total CHO — *negligible*          Total Cals — 415

| | |
|---|---|
| 3 size 3 eggs, hard-boiled and mashed 1 oz (25g) low-fat spread 2 oz (50g) lean boiled ham, chopped finely | Mix all the ingredients together. Chill and use as required. Any excess mixture can be stored for up to 2 days covered in a refrigerator. *Note:* This recipe is *not* suitable for freezing. |

# Cottage Cheese and Apricot Filling

Fills 2 rolls or 1 pitta    Total CHO — 10g    Total Cals — 115

4 oz (100g) reduced-
fat cottage cheese
½ oz (12g) dried
apricots, soaked and
chopped finely

Combine all ingredients well. Chill and use as required.

Note: This recipe is *not* suitable for freezing.

# Sardine, Cucumber and Celery Filling ✓

Fills 2 rolls or 1 pitta    Total CHO — *negligible*    Total Cals — 95

2 oz (50g) sardines in
tomato sauce
1 oz (25g) cucumber,
chopped finely
1 oz (25g) celery,
chopped finely
Dash of tomato sauce

Blend all ingredients well. Chill and use as required.

Note: This recipe is *not* suitable for freezing.

# Spiced Fruit Filling

---

Fills 2 rolls or 1 pitta          Total CHO — 20g          Total Cals — 85

---

*1 small ripe banana,
mashed
2 oz (50g) apple,
chopped finely
1 tablespoon low-fat
natural yogurt
Pinch of ginger*

Mix all ingredients well. Chill and use as required.

*Note:* This recipe freezes well.

---

# Egg and Pepper Filling ✓

---

Fills 2 rolls or 1 pitta    Total CHO — *negligible*    Total Cals — 150

---

*1 egg, hard-boiled and
chopped
1 oz (25g) green
pepper, chopped
Dash of low-calorie
salad cream
Sea salt and freshly
ground black pepper*

Combine all ingredients well. Chill and use as required.

*Note:* This recipe is *not* suitable for freezing.

# Chinese Vegetable Filling

Fills 2 rolls or 1 Pitta        Total CHO — 5g        Total Cals — 10

*2 oz (50g)
beansprouts, chopped
roughly
1 oz (25g) red pepper,
chopped
1 oz (25g)
mushrooms, chopped
Dash of soy sauce*

Mix all ingredients well. Chill and use as required.

*Note:* This recipe needs to be used the day it is made. It is *not* suitable for freezing.

# Cheesy Corn Filling

Fills 4 large rolls or 3 pittas
Total CHO — 65g        Total Cals — 600

*8 oz (225g) reduced-
fat cottage cheese
6 spring onions,
chopped
1×11 oz (300g) tin
sweetcorn
Sea salt and freshly
ground black pepper
2 size 3 eggs, hard-
boiled and chopped*

Combine all ingredients well. Chill and use as required.

*Note:* This recipe is *not* suitable for freezing.

# Beef 'n' Bean Round Filling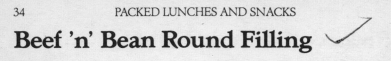

---

Makes 12     Total CHO — 50g     Total Cals — 1080

---

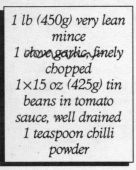

*1 lb (450g) very lean
mince
1 clove garlic, finely
chopped
1×15 oz (425g) tin
beans in tomato
sauce, well drained
1 teaspoon chilli
powder*

**1.** Mix all ingredients well until smooth.
**2.** Shape into 12 rounds. Place on a lightly
oiled baking sheet and bake at
400°F/200°C (Gas Mark 6) for 15 minutes.
Place on crumpled kitchen paper (to
absorb excess fat) until cool. Use as
required.

Each round contains 4g CHO and 90
calories.

*Note:* This recipe freezes well wrapped
individually.

---

# Fillings Using Reduced-fat
# Hard Cheese

# Reduced-fat Cheese and Chives √

---

Fills 3 large rolls or 2 pittas
Total CHO — 5g          Total Cals — 270

---

*4 oz (100g) reduced-
fat cheese, grated
2 oz (50g) chives*

Mix ingredients together. Chill and use as
required.

---

# Reduced-fat Cheese and Cucumber

Fills 3 large rolls or 2 pittas
Total CHO — *negligible*          Total Cals — 260

*4 oz (100g) reduced-fat cheese, grated*
*¼ cucumber*

Mix ingredients together. Chill and use as required.

# Reduced-fat Cheese and Pineapple

Fills 3 large rolls or 2 pittas
Total CHO — 8g          Total Cals — 280

*4 oz (100g) reduced-fat cheese, grated*
*2 oz (50g) pineapple (tinned in natural juice), drained*

Mix ingredients together. Chill and use as required.

*Note:* All these recipes freeze well. Any excess mixture can be stored for up to 2 days covered in a refrigerator.

# Mushroom Quark Filling

Fills 4 large rolls *or* 3 pittas
Total CHO — 5g          Total Cals — 110

2 oz (50g)
mushrooms, very
finely chopped
3 oz (75g) quark
cheese
1 tablespoon low-fat
natural yogurt
Seasoning to taste

Blend all ingredients together well (preferably using a food processor or electric blender). Chill and use as required.

*Note:* This recipe is *not* suitable for freezing.

# Cheese, Apple and Peanut Filling

Fills 4 large rolls *or* 3 pittas
Total CHO — 30g          Total Cals — 630

4 oz (100g) reduced-
fat hard cheese, grated
2 eating apples,
chopped
2 oz (50g) peanuts,
chopped

Mix all ingredients well. Chill and use as required.

*Note:* This recipe is *not* suitable for freezing.

# Sardine Tomato Filling

Fills 4 large rolls *or* 3 pittas
Total CHO — *negligible*      Total Cals — 230

1×4 oz (100g) tin
sardines in tomato
sauce
1 tablespoon tomato
purée
1 tablespoon grated
horseradish
½ teaspoon lemon
juice
2 tablespoons low-fat
natural yogurt

Blend all ingredients together well. Chill and use as required.

*Note:* This recipe is *not* suitable for freezing.

# Curried Corn Filling ✓

Fills 4 large rolls *or* 3 pittas
Total CHO — 10g      Total Cals — 190

4 oz (100g) reduced-
fat soft cheese
3 oz (75g) sweetcorn
½ teaspoon curry
powder

Mix all ingredients well. Chill and use as required.

*Note:* This recipe is *not* suitable for freezing.

# Corn, Pepper and Bean Sprout

Fills 4 large rolls *or* 3 pittas
Total CHO — 25g          Total Cals — 145

*4 oz (100g)
beansprouts
2 oz (50g)
mushrooms, chopped
8 radishes, sliced
1 small carrot, grated
3 oz (75g) sweetcorn
1 small green pepper,
deseeded and chopped
1 tablespoon low-fat
natural yogurt*

Mix all ingredients together well. Chill and use as required.

*Note:* This recipe is *not* suitable for freezing.

# Mackerel Cheese

Fills 4 large rolls *or* 3 pittas
Total CHO — 5g          Total Cals — 235

*1×4 oz (100g) tin
mackerel in tomato
sauce
1 tablespoon low-fat
natural yogurt
3 oz (75g) quark
cheese
Seasoning to taste
1 teaspoon lemon
juice*

Blend all ingredients together well (preferably using a food processor or electric blender). Chill and use as required.

*Note:* This recipe is *not* suitable for freezing.

# Curried Egg Filling ✓

---

Fills 4 large rolls *or* 3 pittas
Total CHO — *negligible*          Total Cals — 325

---

4 size 3 eggs, hard-
boiled and mashed
Paprika pepper
1 teaspoon curry
powder
2 tablespoons low-
calorie salad cream

Mix all ingredients well (preferably in a food processor). Chill and use as required.

Note: This recipe is *not* suitable for freezing.

---

# Waldorf Cheese Filling

---

Fills 4 large rolls *or* 3 pittas
Total CHO — 10g          Total Cals — 240

---

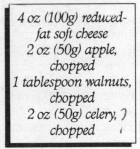

4 oz (100g) reduced-
fat soft cheese
2 oz (50g) apple,
chopped
1 tablespoon walnuts,
chopped
2 oz (50g) celery,
chopped

Mix all ingredients well. Chill and use as required.

Note: This recipe is *not* suitable for freezing.

# Beef, Yogurt and Onion Filling

Fills 4 large rolls *or* 3 pittas
Total CHO — 15g          Total Cals — 330

2 oz (50g) *reduced-fat hard cheese, grated*
3 oz (75g) very *lean mince, cooked, skimmed and cooled*
2 oz (50g) *potato, cooked, cooled and cubed*
2 oz (50g) *onion, chopped finely*
2 tablespoons *low-fat natural yogurt*

Mix all ingredients well, removing as much fat as possible from the cooked mince. Chill and use as required.

*Note:* This recipe is *not* suitable for freezing.

# Quarky Peanut Butter Filling

Fills 4 large rolls *or* 3 pittas
Total CHO — 10g          Total Cals — 275

2 tablespoons *peanut butter*
3 oz (75g) *quark cheese*
1 tablespoon *low-fat natural yogurt*
*Sea salt and freshly ground black pepper*

Blend all ingredients together well (preferably using a food processor or electric blender). Chill and use as required.

*Note:* This recipe is *not* suitable for freezing.

# Small 'n' Speedy Potato Wholemeal Rolls

Makes 10    Total CHO — 150g    Total Cals — 740

*6 oz (175g) wholemeal
self-raising flour
3 oz (75g) potato,
cooked, mashed, cold
1 size 3 egg
¼ pint (150ml)
skimmed milk*

**1.** Mix the flour, potato and egg. Gradually add milk until a smooth dough is formed.
**2.** Divide into 10 and roll into balls. Place on a lightly oiled baking tray. Bake at 400°F/200°C (Gas Mark 6) for 25-30 minutes until golden brown and hollow sounding when tapped. Allow to cool on a wire rack.

Each roll contains 15g CHO and 75 calories.

*Note:* This recipe freezes well.

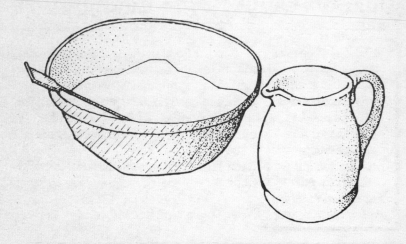

# Small 'n' Speedy Wholemeal Rolls

Makes 8          Total CHO — 160g          Total Cals — 860

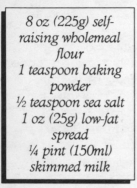

*8 oz (225g) self-raising wholemeal flour*
*1 teaspoon baking powder*
*½ teaspoon sea salt*
*1 oz (25g) low-fat spread*
*¼ pint (150ml) skimmed milk*

**1.** Mix the flour, baking powder and salt. Rub in the low-fat spread. Add milk and mix to a smooth dough. Turn out onto a floured board and knead for 5 minutes.
**2.** Divide into 8 and shape as required. Place on a lightly oiled baking tray and glaze with a little milk. Bake at 425°F/220°C (Gas Mark 7) for 15 minutes. Allow to cool on a wire rack.

Each roll contains 20g CHO and 110 calories.

*Note:* This recipe freezes well.

# Bran Muffins

Makes 18          Total CHO — 190g          Total Cals — 1290

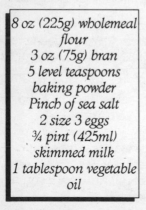

*8 oz (225g) wholemeal flour*
*3 oz (75g) bran*
*5 level teaspoons baking powder*
*Pinch of sea salt*
*2 size 3 eggs*
*¾ pint (425ml) skimmed milk*
*1 tablespoon vegetable oil*

**1.** Mix the flour, bran, baking powder and salt. Beat together the eggs, milk and oil. Add to flour mixture. Mix gently.
**2.** Fill 18 lightly oiled deep bun tins. Bake at 425°F/220°C (Gas Mark 7) for 15 minutes. Allow to cool on a wire rack.

Each muffin contains 10g CHO and 70 calories.

*Note:* This recipe freezes well.

# 3. Pancakes, Pastries and Flans

*Lots of alternatives to sandwiches*

## Pancake Parcels

| Makes 8 | Total CHO — 80g | Total Cals — 485 |
|---------|-----------------|------------------|

*4 oz (100g) wholemeal flour*
*A pinch of sea salt*
*1 size 3 egg, beaten*
*½ pint (275ml) skimmed milk*

**1.** Beat all ingredients together well until a smooth batter is formed. Leave to stand for 30 minutes.

**2.** Heat a little oil in a heavy based pan. Pour a little batter into the pan. After 3-4 minutes turn and cook other side. Allow to cool, stack — separated by layers of greaseproof paper.

Fill as desired — three suggested fillings are given here. *Remember* to add filling figures to pancake figures.

Each pancake contains 10g CHO and 60 calories.

*Note:* These pancakes freeze well empty — separated by layers of greaseproof paper. Check your chosen filling to see if you can freeze the filled parcel.

# Fruit Salad and Lemon Pancake Filling

Fills 10 pancakes     Total CHO — 250g     Total Cals — 950

5 oz (150g) dried
prunes
5 oz (150g) dried
apricots
5 oz (150g) sultanas
6 fl oz (200ml) orange
juice
Rind of a lemon,
grated

**1.** Soak dried fruit overnight in orange juice.
**2.** Stone the prunes and add the lemon rind. Simmer gently for approximately 10 minutes until liquid is thick and syrupy. Leave to cool.

*Note:* This recipe freezes well.

# Spicy Apple Pancake Filling ✓

Fills 8 pancakes     Total CHO — 40g     Total Cals — 180

1 lb (450g) cooking
apples, peeled and
diced
4 fl oz (100ml) orange
juice
1 teaspoon lemon
juice
1 teaspoon mixed
spice
Liquid sweetener to
taste

Cook apples in fruit juices and spice for 15-20 minutes until the apple is of a thick sauce consistency. Leave to cool and add sweetener to taste.

*Note:* This recipe freezes well.

# Kipper and Cheese Pancake Filling

Fills 8 pancakes     Total CHO — 10g     Total Cals — 520

8 oz (225g) cooked
flaked kipper or
mackerel (smoked)
4 oz (100g) cottage
cheese
1 medium onion,
finely chopped
Sea salt and freshly
ground black pepper
1 tablespoon fresh
chopped parsley
1 tablespoon lemon
juice

Combine all ingredients thoroughly.

Note: This recipe is *not* suitable for freezing.

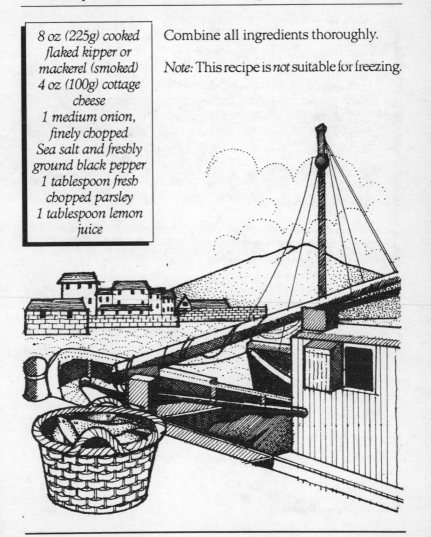

# Lentil Tuna Loaf

Slices into 8     Total CHO — 135g     Total Cals — 1100

8 oz (225g) lentils,
soaked overnight
1 onion, chopped
finely
2 oz (50g) reduced-
fat hard cheese, grated
¼ pint (150ml) low-fat
natural yogurt
2 teaspoons dried sage
4 oz (100g) tuna in
brine, drained and
flaked
1 size 3 egg, beaten
Sea salt and freshly
ground black pepper

**1.** Simmer the lentils for 30 minutes and then drain.

**2.** Mix all ingredients well ensuring even distribution of egg and yogurt.

**3.** Press the mixture into a lightly oiled 2 lb (900g) loaf tin. Bake at 400°F/200°C (Gas Mark 6) for about 1 hour or until firm to the touch. Allow to cool in the tin.

Each slice contains about 15g CHO and 140 calories.

Note: This recipe freezes well. Wrap individual slices and freeze for easy packing.

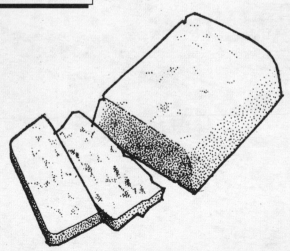

# Stripy Chicken and Lentil Loaf

Slices into 10    Total CHO — 140g    Total Cals — 1120

*4 oz (100g) green lentils, soaked overnight*
*4 oz (100g) orange lentils, soaked overnight*
*1 onion, finely chopped*
*2 oz (50g) reduced-fat hard cheese, grated*
*¼ pint (150ml) low-fat natural yogurt*
*4 oz (100g) chicken, cooked and finely chopped*
*1 size 3 egg beaten*
*Sea salt and freshly ground black pepper*

**1.** Simmer the lentils *separately* for 30 minutes and then drain.
**2.** Place green lentils in one bowl and orange lentils in another.
**3.** Mix all remaining ingredients — add half of this mixture to each set of lentils and mix well.
**4.** Press alternating layers of the green and orange mixture into a lightly oiled 2 lb (900g) loaf tin.
**5.** Bake at 400°F/200°C (Gas Mark 6) for about 1 hour or until firm to the touch. Allow to cool in the tin.

Each slice contains about 15g CHO and 110 calories.

*Note:* This recipe freezes well. Wrap individual slices and freeze for easy packing.

# Cheesy Snacks

Makes 10      Total CHO — 50g      Total Cals — 650

2 oz (50g) low-fat spread
3 oz (75g) reduced-fat cheese, grated
1 teaspoon French mustard (optional)
2 oz (50g) wholemeal flour
2 oz (50g) All-Bran, crushed, or Bran Buds

**1.** Beat the low-fat spread, cheese and mustard together. Add the flour and bran and mix well together.

**2.** Form into walnut sized pieces and place on a lightly oiled baking tray. Flatten with a damp fork. Bake at 350°F/180°C (Gas Mark 4) for 12 minutes. Allow to cool on a wire rack.

Each snack contains 5g CHO and 65 calories.

*Note:* This recipe freezes well.

# Mushroom Loaf

Slices into 4      Total CHO — 20g      Total Cals — 480

1 onion, diced
1 green pepper, deseeded and diced
3 oz (75g) mushrooms
1 oz (25g) wholemeal breadcrumbs
1 size 3 egg
3 oz (75g) reduced-fat hard cheese
Mixed herbs
Garlic salt

**1.** Fry the onion and pepper in a little oil until tender. Add mushrooms. Turn off heat, add breadcrumbs and egg.

**2.** Turn into a lightly oiled 1 lb (450g) loaf tin. Press in well, sprinkle with seasonings and grated cheese.

**3.** Bake at 350°F/180°C (Gas Mark 4) for 20 minutes. Allow to cool in the tin.

Each portion contains 5g CHO and 120 calories.

*Note:* This recipe is *not* suitable for freezing.

# Fluffy Vegetable Bake

---

Serves 5          Total CHO — 25g          Total Cals — 750

---

**Vegetable Set (1)**
*2 medium sized
aubergines, sliced
2 tablespoons
vegetable oil
2 size 3 eggs,
separated
1×5 oz (150g) carton
low-fat natural yogurt
Sea salt and freshly
ground black pepper*

**Vegetable Set (2)**
*5 carrots, sliced
2 size 3 eggs,
separated
1×5 oz (150g) carton
low-fat natural yogurt*

**Set 1**

**1.** Sprinkle aubergines with salt — cover and leave for 2 hours. Rinse in cold water and chop finely.

**2.** Sauté in oil until soft. Allow to cool, stir in egg yolks and yogurt, salt and pepper. Reserve.

**Set 2**

**1.** Boil carrots in salted water until tender. Drain. Mash and add the egg yolks and natural yogurt.

**2.** Whisk all egg whites. Fold half into each vegetable mixture.

Place alternating layers of the vegetable sets in a lightly oiled 2 lb (900g) loaf tin. Bake at 375°F/190°C (Gas Mark 5) for 1 hour or until set. Allow to cool in the tin.

Each portion contains 5g CHO and 150 calories.

*Note:* This recipe is *not* suitable for freezing.

# Wholemeal Vegetable Pastries ✓

Makes 12     Total CHO — 250g     Total Cals — 1470

### Pastry
3 oz (75g) low-fat
spread
3 oz (75g) white
vegetable fat
12 oz (350g)
wholemeal flour

### Sauce
1 oz (25g) low-fat
spread
1 oz (25g) wholemeal
flour
¼ pint (150ml)
skimmed milk
1 oz (25g) reduced-
fat hard cheese, grated

### Filling
1 carrot, grated
1 parsnip, grated
1 leek, grated
1 courgette, finely
chopped

**1.** Rub the fat into the flour, mix to a smooth dough with a little cold water. Divide into 12.

**2.** Roll each portion to a 3 in (7cm) circle. Place on a baking tray and chill.

**3.** Place all sauce ingredients in a pan. Bring to the boil, stir, simmer for 2 minutes.

**4.** Add enough sauce to the vegetables to just dampen them. Divide the vegetables between the circles. Brush the edges with beaten egg and seal by folding over. Brush with beaten egg.

**5.** Bake at 400°F/200°C (Gas Mark 6) for 30-35 minutes. Allow to cool on a wire rack.

Each pastry contains 20g CHO and 120 calories.

*Note:* This recipe freezes well.

120
Cals

# Individual Flans

Makes 8     Total CHO — 150g     Total Cals — 1530

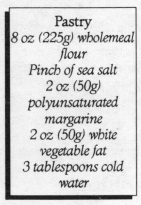

### Pastry
*8 oz (225g) wholemeal
flour
Pinch of sea salt
2 oz (50g)
polyunsaturated
margarine
2 oz (50g) white
vegetable fat
3 tablespoons cold
water*

**1.** Mix the flour and salt together. Rub in the margarine and vegetable fat. Mix in the water to form a soft pastry. Allow to relax in the refrigerator for 15 minutes.
**2.** Line 8 individual flan rings. Bake blind at 425°F/220°C (Gas Mark 7) for 15-20 minutes.

# White Sauce

Makes 1 pint     Total CHO — 45g     Total Cals — 365

*1 oz (25g) low-fat
spread
1 oz (25g) wholemeal
flour
1 pint (550ml)
skimmed milk*

**1.** Melt the low-fat spread gently. Stir in the flour to a smooth paste.
**2.** Gradually add the milk — stirring all the time. Bring to the boil, simmer for 2 minutes. Use as required.

# Tuna and Cucumber Filling  ✓

Filling — enough for 8 cases
Total CHO — 25g          Total Cals — 415

1 × 7 oz (200g) tin
tuna in brine
½ cucumber
½ pint (275ml) White
Sauce (see
page 51)

**1.** Make up basic white sauce. Add flaked tuna and cubed cucumber (reserving 4 rings for decoration). Pour into flan tins. Decorate with cucumber rings.

# Sweetcorn and Pepper Filling

Filling — enough for 8 cases
Total CHO — 55g          Total Cals — 320

1 small tin sweetcorn,
drained
1 green pepper
½ pint (275ml) White
Sauce (see page 51)

**1.** Make up basic White Sauce. Add sweetcorn and cubed pepper (reserving 4 rings to decorate). Pour into flan tins. Decorate with pepper rings.

Note: All of these recipes freeze well.

N.B. Remember to add base and filling figures together.

# Curried Vegetable Quiche ✓

---

Serves 8     Total CHO — 160g     Total Cals — 1160

---

### Pastry
3 oz (75g) low-fat
spread
6 oz (175g) 81% self-
raising flour
Pinch of sea salt

### Filling
1 leek, chopped finely
1 carrot, grated
1 onion, grated
2 size 3 eggs
½ pint (275ml)
skimmed milk
2 teaspoons curry
powder
Sea salt and freshly
ground black pepper

**1.** Make the pastry by rubbing the fat into the flour and salt. Bring to a smooth dough with enough water to bind. Roll out and line an 8 in (20cm) flan ring. Allow to relax in the refrigerator for 15 minutes.

**2.** Bake blind at 400°F/200°C (Gas Mark 6) for 10 minutes until set and golden brown.

**3.** Sprinkle vegetables into base. Mix egg, milk and seasoning, pour into ring. Bake at 400°F/200°C (Gas Mark 6) for 20-30 minutes. Allow to cool in the ring.

Each slice contains 20g CHO and 145 calories.

*Note:* This recipe freezes well.

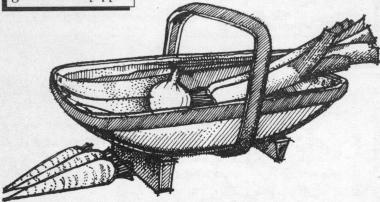

# Tuna and Spinach Quiche

Serves 8      Total CHO — 120g      Total Cals — 1480

### Pastry
3 oz (75g)
polyunsaturated
margarine
6 oz (175g) self-
raising wholemeal
flour
Sea salt
Cold water to bind

### Filling
2 size 3 eggs
¼ pint (150ml)
skimmed milk
Sea salt and freshly
ground black pepper
8 oz (225g) spinach —
cooked and drained
4 oz (100g) tin tuna
in brine, drained

1. Make pastry by rubbing fat into flour and salt. Bring to a soft dough with cold water. Roll out and line an 8 in (20cm) flan ring. Allow to relax in fridge for 15 minutes.
2. Meanwhile beat together the eggs, milk and seasoning. Place the spinach and tuna in the base and pour on egg mixture.
3. Bake at 400°F/200°C (Gas Mark 6) for 20 minutes. Allow to cool in the ring.

Each portion contains 15g CHO and 185 calories.

Note: This recipe freezes well.

# Tuna and Tomato Flan      ✓

Serves 8      Total CHO — 140g      Total Cals — 1520

### Pastry
3 oz (75g)
polyunsaturated
margarine
6 oz (175g) 81% self-
raising flour
Sea salt
Water to bind

1. Make pastry by rubbing margarine into flour and salt. Bring to a soft dough with cold water. Roll out and line an 8 in (20cm) flan ring. Allow to relax in the refrigerator for 15 minutes.
2. Mix the tuna, tomatoes and onion. Place in the flan case. Beat eggs, milk and seasoning and pour into the case.

**Filling**
1×7 oz (200g) tin
tuna in brine, drained
1×14 oz (400g) tin
tomatoes, drained and
chopped
1 onion, chopped
1 size 3 egg
¼ pint (150ml)
skimmed milk
Sea salt and freshly
ground black pepper

**3.** Bake at 375°F/190°C (Gas Mark 5) for 30-40 minutes. Allow to cool in the ring.

Each portion contains about 20g CHO and 190 calories.

*Note:* This recipe freezes well.

# Cottage Leek Quiche

Slices into 8     Total CHO — 160g     Total Cals — 1230

**Pastry**
3 oz (75g) low-fat
spread
6 oz (175g) 81% self-
raising flour
Pinch of sea salt
Water to bind

**Filling**
2 leeks, washed and
thinly sliced
1×7 oz (200g) tin
sweetcorn
4 oz (100g) cottage
cheese
1 egg, separated
Sea salt and freshly
ground black pepper

**1.** Make the pastry by rubbing the fat into the flour and salt. Bring to a soft dough with enough water to bind. Line an 8 in (20cm) flan ring. Allow to relax in the refrigerator for 15 minutes.
**2.** Bake blind at 400°F/200°C (Gas Mark 6) for 10 minutes. Place leeks and sweetcorn in base.
**3.** Mix cheese and egg yolk well. Whisk egg white. Gently fold egg white into yolk mixture. Pour over vegetables.
**4.** Bake at 350°F/180°C (Gas Mark 4) for 35 minutes until springy to the touch. Allow to cool in the ring.

Each slice contains 20g CHO and 155 calories.

*Note:* Raw pastry case freezes well. The completed quiche can be satisfactorily frozen by wrapping each portion separately.

# Spiced Bean Pie

Serves 5          Total CHO — 125g          Total Cals — 1300

### Pastry
2 oz (50g) low-fat
spread
4 oz (100g) wholemeal
flour
Water to bind

### Filling
1 onion, diced
½ oz (15g) low-fat
spread for frying
8 oz (225g) very lean
mince
½ teaspoon chilli
powder
1 teaspoon turmeric
Seasoning to taste
1 tablespoon tomato
purée
⅛ pint (75ml) beef
stock
1 tablespoon soy sauce
2 oz (50g) aduki
beans, soaked
overnight and cooked*
1×7 oz (200g) tin
baked beans

**1.** Make pastry by rubbing fat into flour. Bring to a soft dough with water.

**2.** Roll out and line a 6 in (15cm) flan ring. Allow to relax in the refrigerator for 15 minutes.

**3.** Bake blind at 425°F/220°C (Gas Mark 7) for 20 minutes.

**4.** Fry the onion, mince, then add rest of ingredients. Simmer for 30 minutes, stirring occasionally.

**5.** Fill flan case with meat mixture. Bake in a moderate oven for 15 minutes. Allow to cool in the ring.

Each serving contains 25g CHO and 260 calories.

*Note:* This recipe freezes well.

*Boiled for 1 hour or pressure cooked for 15 minutes.

# Macaroni and Fish Flan

Serves 8      Total CHO — 160g      Total Cals — 1560

### Pastry
3 oz (75g) low-fat
spread
6 oz (175g) self-raising
wholemeal flour
Sea salt
Cold water to bind

### Filling
2 size 3 eggs
¼ pint (150ml)
skimmed milk
Sea salt and freshly
ground black pepper
4 oz (100g) kipper
fillet, cooked and
flaked
2 oz (50g) wholegrain
macaroni, cooked and
drained
2 oz (50g) reduced-fat
hard cheese
1 onion, chopped

**1.** Make pastry by rubbing fat into flour and salt. Bring to a soft dough with cold water. Roll out and line an 8 in (20cm) flan ring. Allow to relax in the refrigerator for 15 minutes.

**2.** Meanwhile beat together the eggs, milk and seasoning. Mix the fish, pasta, onion and cheese. Place in the base. Pour on the egg mixture.

**3.** Bake at 400°F/200°C (Gas Mark 6) for 20 minutes. Allow to cool in the ring.

Each portion contains 20g CHO and 195 calories.

*Note:* This recipe freezes well.

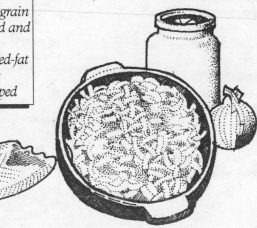

# Lentil Cheese Slice

Slices into 10    Total CHO — 150g    Total Cals — 1250

### Pastry
2 oz (50g) low-fat spread
5 oz (150g) self-raising wholemeal flour
Pinch of sea salt
Water to bind

### Filling
4 oz (100g) lentils — soaked for 4 hours and cooked for 10 minutes
1 large onion, chopped
2 oz (50g) reduced-fat cottage cheese
1 size 3 egg
Sea salt and freshly ground black pepper
2 oz (50g) reduced-fat hard cheese, grated

**1.** Make pastry by rubbing fat into flour and salt. Bring to a soft dough with enough water to bind. Roll out to line an 8 in (20cm) square tin. Allow to relax in the refrigerator for 15 minutes.

**2.** Mix the lentils and onion. Beat the cottage cheese and egg together. Add to the lentil mixture and season. Place in pastry case. Sprinkle on grated cheese.

**3.** Bake at 400°F/200°C (Gas Mark 6) for 30 minutes. Allow to cool in the tin.

Each slice contains 15g CHO and 125 calories.

*Note:* This recipe freezes well.

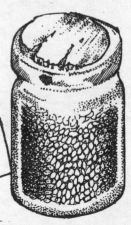

# Tomato, Cheese Flan

Serves 8      Total CHO — 160g      Total Cals — 1680

### Pastry
3 oz (75g) low-fat
spread
6 oz (175g) 81% self-
raising flour
Pinch of sea salt
Water to bind

### Filling
1×15 oz (425g) tin
tomatoes, chopped
3 medium onions,
chopped
2 tablespoons
vegetable oil
Mixed herbs
French mustard
2 size 3 eggs
½ pint (275ml)
skimmed milk
Sea salt and freshly
ground black pepper
3 oz (75g) reduced-
fat hard cheese, grated

1.  Make pastry by rubbing fat into flour and salt. Bring to a soft dough with cold water. Roll out and line an 8 in (20cm) flan ring. Allow to relax in the refrigerator for 15 minutes.

2.  Meanwhile drain and chop tomatoes. Gently sauté the onions in oil for 10 minutes. Add herbs and mustard to taste to the tomatoes. Mix the eggs, milk, salt and pepper.

3.  Spread onions in base. Cover with tomato mixture. Pour on egg mixture. Sprinkle with cheese.

4.  Bake at 400°F/200°C (Gas Mark 6) for 30-40 minutes until set and golden brown. Allow to cool in the ring.

Each slice contains 20g CHO and 210 calories.

Note: The raw pastry case freezes well.

# Creamy Lemon Flan  ✓

---

Serves 8     Total CHO — 110g     Total Cals — 1250

---

**Base**
3 oz (75g) crunch
bars, e.g. Jordans
2 oz (50g) All-Bran
or Bran Buds
2 oz (50g) low-fat
spread

**Topping**
6 oz (175g) reduced-
fat soft cheese
3 eggs, separated
Juice and rind of
1 lemon
2 teaspoons clear
honey
2 oz (50g) sultanas

**1.** Crush up the crunch bars and bran together with the end of a rolling pin.
**2.** Melt the fat and gently stir in the bran and bars until coated. Press into a lightly oiled 8 in (20cm) flan ring.
**3.** Beat the low-fat cheese with egg yolks, lemon rind and juice. Stir in honey and sultanas. Whisk egg whites until firm and fold into cheese mixture.
**4.** Pour the cheese mixture into the flan case. Bake at 350°F/180°C (Gas Mark 4) for 15 minutes and then 300°F/150°C (Gas Mark 2) for 10 minutes. Allow to cool in the ring.

Each slice contains about 15g CHO and 160 calories.

*Note:* This recipe is *not* suitable for freezing.

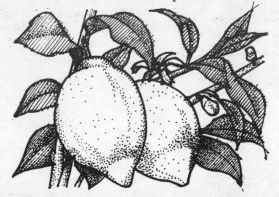

# Peach Yogurt Slice

Serves 10    Total CHO — 100g    Total Cals — 900

### Base
2 oz (50g) low-fat spread
4 oz (100g) wholemeal flour
Pinch of sea salt
4 teaspoons cold water

### Topping
5 oz (150g) reduced-fat soft cheese
1×5 oz (150g) carton low-fat natural yogurt
8 oz (225g) peach slices in natural juice, drained (reserve juice)
1 lemon, rind and juice
¼ oz (5g) ½ sachet gelatine

1. Rub fat into flour and salt and add water. Roll out and line square 8 in (20cm) tin. Allow to relax in the refrigerator for 15 minutes. Bake blind at 350°F/180°C (Gas Mark 4) for 20 minutes. Leave to cool in the tin.

2. Mix cheese and yogurt and mash up the fruit (reserving 4 peach slices). Stir in grated lemon rind. Melt gelatine in heated, but *not* boiling, peach juice. Allow to cool until almost set. Whisk into cheese mixture.

3. Fill the case and leave to set in the refrigerator. Decorate when firm with peach slices.

Each slice contains 10g CHO and 90 calories.

*Note:* This recipe is *not* suitable for freezing, although the raw case freezes well.

# Autumn Apple Slices ✓

Makes 18     Total CHO — 180g     Total Cals — 1670

---

*4 oz (100g)
polyunsaturated
margarine
6 oz (175g) self-
raising wholemeal
flour
12 oz (350g) cooking
apple, peeled, chopped
and puréed
3 oz (75g) raisins
1 oz (25g) hazel-nuts
1 teaspoon cinnamon*

**1.** Rub fat into flour and knead until it starts to come together. Press mixture into a lightly oiled, shallow swiss roll tin.

**2.** Mix the puréed apple, raisins, nuts and cinnamon. Spread onto base. Bake at 400°F/200°C (Gas Mark 6) for 40 minutes. Allow to cool slightly. Cut and allow to cool on a wire rack.

Each slice contains 10g CHO and 95 calories.

*Note:* This recipe is *not* suitable for freezing.

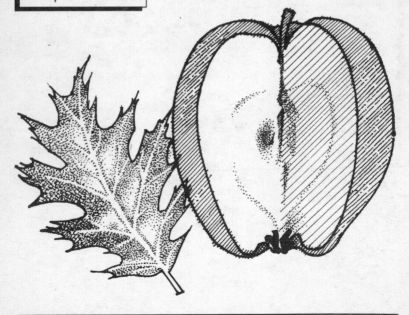

# Pineapple and Cheese Quiche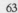

Serves 8      Total CHO — 160g      Total Cals — 1520

### Pastry
*3 oz (75g)
polyunsaturated
margarine
6 oz (175g) 81% self-
raising flour
Sea salt
Cold water to bind*

### Filling
*1×14 oz (400g) tin
pineapple in natural
juice, drained and
chopped finely
5 oz (150g) reduced-
fat cottage cheese
2 size 3 eggs,
separated*

**1.** Make pastry by rubbing fat into flour and salt. Bring to a soft dough with cold water. Roll out and line an 8 in (20cm) flan ring. Allow to relax in the refrigerator for 15 minutes.

**2.** Mix the pineapple, cheese and egg yolks. Whisk the egg whites to stiff peaks. Carefully fold into pineapple mixture. Pour immediately into pastry case.

**3.** Bake at 400°F/200°C (Gas Mark 6) for 20 minutes. Allow to cool in ring.

Each portion contains 20g CHO and 190 calories.

*Note:* This recipe is not suitable for freezing although the raw base freezes well.

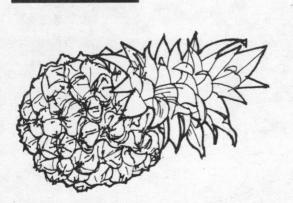

# 4. Fruit and Vegetables

*A good way to add crunch to a lunch box*

## Pepper, Radish and Corn Salad

| Serves 6 | Total CHO — 30g | Total Cals — 180 |
|---|---|---|

*8 oz (225g)
beansprouts
3 oz (75g)
mushrooms, chopped
8 radishes, sliced
1 medium carrot,
grated
5 oz (150g) sweetcorn
1 green pepper,
deseeded and chopped
2 tablespoons wine
vinegar*

Toss all ingredients well. Chill before serving.

Each portion contains 5g CHO and 30 calories.

*Note:* This recipe is *not* suitable for freezing but will store overnight in the refrigerator.

# Wholewheat Pasta Salad

4 large portions    Total CHO — 80g    Total Cals — 400

4 oz (100g)
wholewheat pasta
shells
2 medium carrots,
sliced
1 medium green
pepper, deseeded and
chopped
4 stalks celery,
trimmed and chopped
½ teaspoon garlic
powder
1 tablespoon Worcester
sauce
Fresh parsley, chopped

**1.** Put pasta in a pan of boiling water and cook for 15-20 minutes. Drain and leave to cool.

**2.** Mix with the remaining ingredients and garnish with chopped parsley

Each portion contains 20g CHO and 00 calories.

*Note:* This recipe is *not* suitable for freezing.

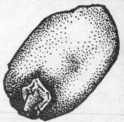

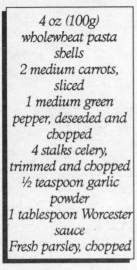

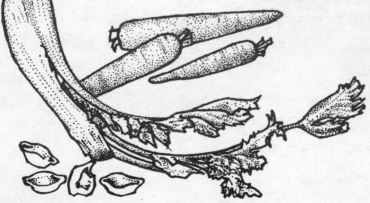

# Beany Coleslaw    ✓

---

Serves 2    Total CHO — 30g    Total Cals — 170

---

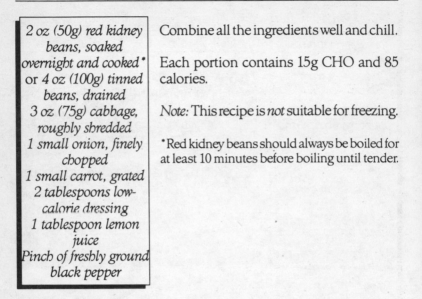

2 oz (50g) red kidney
beans, soaked
overnight and cooked*
or 4 oz (100g) tinned
beans, drained
3 oz (75g) cabbage,
roughly shredded
1 small onion, finely
chopped
1 small carrot, grated
2 tablespoons low-
calorie dressing
1 tablespoon lemon
juice
Pinch of freshly ground
black pepper

Combine all the ingredients well and chill.

Each portion contains 15g CHO and 85 calories.

Note: This recipe is not suitable for freezing.

*Red kidney beans should always be boiled for at least 10 minutes before boiling until tender.

# Crunchy Bean Salad

---

Serves 5    Total CHO — 75g    Total Cals — 600

---

3 oz (75g) soya beans,
soaked
3 oz (75g) red kidney
beans, soaked
3 oz (75g) French
green beans, blanched

1. Simmer the soya beans for 3 hours or pressure cook for 45 minutes. Leave to cool.
2. Boil red kidney beans for at least 10 minutes and then simmered for one hour. Leave to cool.
3. Mix all the ingredients together in one bowl. Chill.

8 oz (225g) white
cabbage, shredded
3 tablespoons low-fat
natural yogurt
½ teaspoon celery salt

Each serving contains 15g CHO and 120 calories.

Note: This recipe is *not* suitable for freezing.

# Pasta and Bean Salad

Serves 8      Total CHO — 200g      Total Cals — 960

7 oz (200g)
wholewheat pasta
shells
1×7 oz (200g) tin red
kidney beans, drained
1×7 oz (200g) tin
butter beans, drained
2 medium carrots,
grated
1 small spring onion,
chopped
3 tablespoons lemon
juice
Black pepper, to taste
Cayenne pepper, to
taste
Garlic salt, to taste

**1.** Cook the pasta in boiling water for 10 minutes. Drain and cool.
**2.** Place the kidney beans and butter beans in bowl. Add the carrots, onion, pasta and juice. Mix well, season and chill.

Each portion contains 25g CHO and 120 calories.

Note: This recipe is *not* suitable for freezing.

# Spiral Corn Salad

Serves 8        Total CHO — 220g        Total Cals — 1210

8 oz (225g)
wholewheat pasta
spirals
1 large eating apple,
chopped
2 teaspoons lemon
juice
1×6 oz (175g) tin
crab meat, drained
1×11 oz (300g) tin
sweetcorn
Sea salt and freshly
ground black pepper
5 tablespoons low-
calorie salad
cream

**1.** Bring pasta to the boil and simmer until just tender (about 20-30 minutes). Drain well and allow to cool.

**2.** Combine all ingredients well.

Each portion contains about 30g CHO and 150 calories.

*Note:* This recipe is *not* suitable for freezing, but remember you can always do half quantities if you don't want 8 portions. As the portions are large you may only need half a portion.

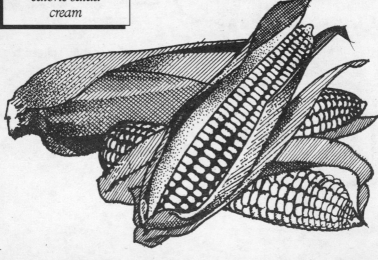

# Concertina Tomato

---

Serves 1          Total CHO — 5g          Total Cals — 220

---

1 large steak tomato
1 hard-boiled egg in 6
slices
2 oz (50g) reduced-
fat hard cheese
2 oz (50g) thinly
sliced cucumber

Dressing
1 tablespoon lemon
juice
1 tablespoon freshly
chopped mint

Chop 6 horizontal slices into the tomato and put a slice of egg in each slice. Cut cheese into 3 slices and cut into 6 triangles. Put a triangle in each slice of the tomato. Put sections of cucumber behind cheese and egg. Sprinkle with dressing.

Note: This recipe is not suitable for freezing.

---

# Orange, Melon and Guavas Salad

---

Serves 4          Total CHO — 60g          Total Cals — 640

---

2 medium oranges,
peeled and sliced
2 large slices of
melon, shaped into
balls
1×10 oz (275g) tin
guavas in natural
juice

Combine all the fruits thoroughly in the juice from the guavas.

Each portion contains 15g CHO and 160 calories.

Note: This recipe is not suitable for freezing.

# Pineapple, Strawberry and Apple Salad

Serves 4        Total CHO — 80g        Total Cals — 320

*1×15 oz (425g) tin pineapple in natural juice*
*1 green skinned dessert apple, sliced and chopped*
*1 tablespoon lemon juice*
*8 oz (225g) fresh strawberries, sliced*

Cut pineapple into bite size pieces. Return to juice and add sliced apple, sprinkled with lemon juice to prevent browning. Finally stir in sliced strawberries.

Each portion contains 20g CHO and 80 calories.

*Note:* This recipe is *not* suitable for freezing.

# Berry Curd Mousse

Serves 6        Total CHO — 30g        Total Cals — 360

*1×10 oz (275g) tin blackberries or raspberries in natural juice*
*8 oz (225g) quark cheese*
*2 sachets* Canderel
*1 sachet gelatine*
*2 tablespoons boiling water*
*2 egg whites, whisked*

**1.** Place fruit (with juice), cheese and *Canderel* into a blender or food processor. Blend until smooth.
**2.** Dissolve gelatine in water and stir into mixture. Fold in the egg whites. Pour into a bowl and leave to set.

Each portion contains 5g CHO and 60 calories.

*Note:* This recipe is *not* suitable for freezing.

# 5. Baked Goods

*Home baking is always popular. These high-fibre, reduced-fat recipes should prove a great success.*

## Muesli Loaf ✓

| Slices into 20 | Total CHO — 400g | Total Cals — 2045 |
| --- | --- | --- |

6 oz (175g) unsweetened muesli
5 oz (150g) sultanas
8 fl oz (250ml) apple juice, unsweetened
Rind of 1 orange
1 large cooking apple, grated
2 oz (50g) low-fat spread
3 oz (75g) wholemeal flour
3 oz (75g) wholemeal self-raising flour
2 teaspoons baking powder
1 teaspoon cinnamon

**1.** Place the muesli and sultanas in the apple juice and leave to soak for ½ hour.
**2.** Add the remaining ingredients and mix well, ensure flour is well mixed in. Spoon into a lightly oiled 2 lb (900g) loaf tin.
**3.** Bake at 350°F/180°C (Gas Mark 4) for 1¾ hours. Allow to cool on a wire rack.

Each portion contains 20g CHO and 100 calories.

*Note:* This recipe freezes well.

# Tropical Tea Bread          ✓

---

Slices into 16     Total CHO — 240g     Total Cals — 2160

---

*4 oz (100g)
polyunsaturated
margarine
2 oz (50g) fructose
(fruit sugar)
2 size 3 eggs
1×14 oz (400g) tin
pineapple in natural
juice, drained and
chopped
4 oz (100g) raisins
3 tablespoons
skimmed milk
8 oz (225g) self-raising
wholemeal flour*

**1.** Cream the margarine and fructose. Beat in the eggs. Add the pineapple, raisins, milk and flour.

**2.** Place in a lightly oiled 2 lb (900g) loaf tin. Bake at 325°F/160°C (Gas Mark 3) for 1-1½ hours. Allow to cool on a wire rack.

Each slice contains 15g CHO and 135 calories.

*Note:* This recipe freezes well.

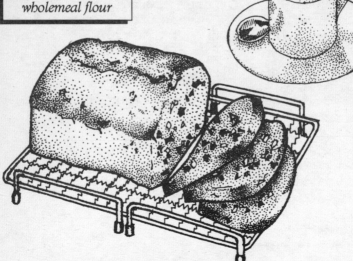

# Wholemeal Apple Sandwich ✓

---

Makes 14 slices     Total CHO — 210g     Total Cals — 1890

---

*4 oz (100g)
polyunsaturated
margarine
4 oz (100g) wholemeal
flour
2 teaspoons baking
powder
6 oz (175g) rolled oats
8 oz (250g) apple,
peeled and chopped
1 size 3 egg*

**1.** Rub the fat into the flour and baking powder. Stir in the oats.

**2.** Heat the apples lightly in a small amount of water. Purée one quarter of the apple and dice the remainder. Mix egg and purée into mixture.

**3.** Divide dough into 2 halves. Roll out both to fit a lightly oiled 7 in (18cm) square tin. Place one square in the tin, cover with remaining apple and then cover with rest of dough.

**4.** Bake at 375°F/190°C (Gas Mark 5) for 20-30 minutes. Allow to cool on a wire rack.

Each slice contains 15g CHO and 135 calories.

*Note:* This recipe freezes well.

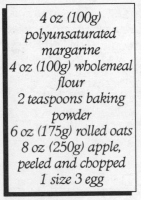
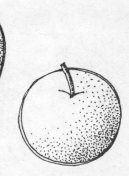

# Gingery Date and Walnut Loaf

Makes 14 slices    Total CHO — 280g    Total Cals — 1820

2 oz (50g) low-fat
spread
8 oz (225g) dried
dates, chopped
2 oz (50g) walnuts,
chopped
A pinch of sea salt
1 teaspoon
bicarbonate of soda
¼ pint (150ml)
boiling water
2 teaspoons dried
ginger
8 oz (225g) 81% self-
raising flour
1 size 3 egg

**1.** Mix the low-fat spread, dates, walnuts, salt and soda. Add water. Mix ginger and flour and stir into mixture. Beat in the egg. Pour into a lightly oiled 1 lb (450g) loaf tin.
**2.** Bake at 325°F/160°C (Gas Mark 3) for 1-1½ hours. Allow to cool in tin. One cold cut into 14.

Each slice contains approximately 20g CHO and 130 calories.

*Note:* This recipe freezes well when wrapped in foil.

# Bran Loaf ✓

Makes 10 slices     Total CHO — 270g     Total Cals — 1250

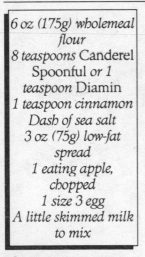

4 oz (100g) All-Bran
6 oz (175g) currants
½ pint (275ml)
   skimmed milk
5 oz (150g) self-raising
   wholemeal flour
16 teaspoons
Canderel Spoonful or
2 teaspoons Diamin

1. Soak the bran and fruit overnight in milk.
2. Add the flour and sweetener. Mix well and place in an oiled 2 lb (900g) loaf tin. Bake at 350°F/180°C (Gas Mark 4) for 1 hour. Allow to cool on a wire rack.

Each slice contains about 30g CHO and 125 calories.

*Note:* This recipe freezes well.

# Wholemeal Apple Cake

Makes 12 slices     Total CHO — 120g     Total Cals — 960

6 oz (175g) wholemeal
   flour
8 teaspoons Canderel
   Spoonful or 1
   teaspoon Diamin
1 teaspoon cinnamon
Dash of sea salt
3 oz (75g) low-fat
   spread
1 eating apple,
   chopped
1 size 3 egg
A little skimmed milk
   to mix

1. Mix the dry ingredients. Add the low-fat spread and apple. Combine with beaten egg and milk.
2. Place in a lightly oiled 1 lb (450g) loaf tin and bake at 375°F/190°C (Gas Mark 5) for 1 hour or until golden brown and firm to the touch.

Each slice contains 10g CHO and 80 calories.

*Note:* This recipe freezes well.

# Fruit Slice ✓

Makes 16 slices     Total CHO — 320g     Total Cals — 2560

### Base
¼ pint (150ml)
boiling water
3 oz (75g) oats
3 oz (75g) self-raising
wholemeal flour
1 oz (25g) desiccated
coconut
⅛ pint (75ml)
vegetable oil

### Filling
¼ pint (150ml)
boiling water
2 oz (50g) raisins,
finely chopped
2 oz (50g) sultanas,
finely chopped
2 oz (50g) currants,
finely chopped
1 large apple
Rind of 1 lemon,
grated

### Topping
3 size 3 eggs
1 oz (25g) fructose
(fruit sugar)
5 oz (150g)
self-raising wholemeal
flour

**1.** Combine all base ingredients together well. Press into a lightly oiled swiss roll tin.
**2.** Mix all filling ingredients together well. Allow to cool slightly. Spread over base.
**3.** Whisk eggs and fructose together until very thick and creamy. Gently fold in the flour. Spread over fruit.
**4.** Bake at 350°F/180°C (Gas Mark 4) for 45 minutes. Allow to cool on a wire rack.

Each slice contains 20g CHO and 160 calories.

*Note:* This recipe freezes well when wrapped in foil.

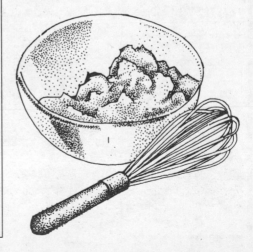

# Date and Apple Baked Slice

Slices into 10     Total CHO — 300g     Total Cals — 1750

**Topping**
4 oz (100g) low-fat
spread
4 oz (100g) wholemeal
flour
3 oz (75g) semolina
2 oz (50g) rolled oats
Grated rind of
1 lemon

**Filling**
6 oz (175g) dates,
chopped
4 tablespoons boiling
water
Juice of 1 lemon
2 large cooking
apples, chopped

**1.** Melt the low-fat spread, stir in the rest of topping ingredients. Press half into the base of a lightly oiled 8 in (20cm) square tin.
**2.** Mix the filling ingredients, allow to cool slightly, pour over the base.
**3.** Top with rest of topping mixture. Press down. Bake at 350°F/180°C (Gas Mark 4) for 40 minutes. Allow to cool in the tin for 10 minutes. Cut and allow to cool on a wire rack.

Each portion contains 30g CHO and 175 calories.

*Note:* This recipe freezes well.

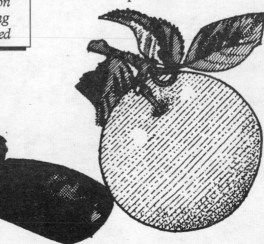

# Bran Banana Bread

Slices into 18    Total CHO — 270g    Total Cals — 2160

6 oz (175g) All-Bran
¼ pint (150ml)
  skimmed milk
3 bananas, mashed
4 oz (100g) low-fat
  spread
2 oz (50g) fructose
  (fruit sugar)
2 size 3 eggs
8 oz (225g) self-
  raising wholemeal
  flour
2 oz (50g) walnuts,
  chopped

**1.** Soak the *All-Bran* in milk for ½ hour. Add the banana. Beat the low-fat spread and fructose together. Beat in the eggs, add the flour and banana mixture. Place in a lightly oiled 2 lb (900g) loaf tin.

**2.** Bake at 350°F/180°C (Gas Mark 4) for 1½ hours. Allow to cool in the tin for 10 minutes and then on a wire rack.

Each slice contains 15g CHO and 120 calories.

*Note:* This recipe freezes well.

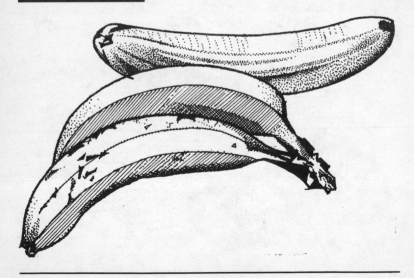

# Date Fingers

---

Makes 10     Total CHO — 100g     Total Cals — 800

---

*1 size 3 egg*
*A pinch of sea salt*
*1 oz (25g)*
*polyunsaturated*
*margarine*
*3 oz (75g) stoned*
*dates, chopped*
*1 oz (25g) walnuts,*
*chopped*
*3 oz (75g) self-raising*
*wholemeal flour*
*½ tablespoon hot*
*water*

**1.** Beat the egg, salt and margarine. Mix in the dates and nuts. Add the flour and water. Mix well. Spread in a lightly oiled 8 in (20cm) square tin.
**2.** Bake at 375°F/190°C (Gas Mark 5) for 20-25 minutes. Allow to cool in tin slightly. Cut into 10. Allow to cool on a wire rack.

Each finger contains 10g CHO and 80 calories.

*Note:* This recipe freezes well.

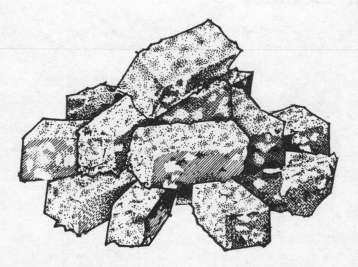

# Fruity Nut Scone Round ✓

Cuts into 8    Total CHO — 200g    Total Cals — 1360

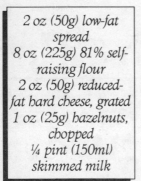

*2 oz (50g) low-fat spread
8 oz (225g) self-raising wholemeal flour
2 oz (50g) sultanas
2 oz (50g) chopped nuts
¼ pint (150ml) skimmed milk*

**1.** Rub the fat into the flour. Stir in the sultanas and nuts. Knead to a soft dough with the milk.
**2.** Shape into a round ¾ in (1½cm) deep. Place on a lightly oiled baking tray. Bake at 425°F/220°C (Gas Mark 7) for 20-25 minutes. Allow to cool on a wire rack.

Each portion contains 25g CHO and 170 calories.

*Note:* This recipe freezes well.

# Cheese and Hazelnut Scones

Makes 16    Total CHO — 160g    Total Cals — 1200

*2 oz (50g) low-fat spread
8 oz (225g) 81% self-raising flour
2 oz (50g) reduced-fat hard cheese, grated
1 oz (25g) hazelnuts, chopped
¼ pint (150ml) skimmed milk*

**1.** Rub the fat into the flour. Add the cheese and nuts. Stir in the milk. Knead to a smooth dough.
**2.** Roll out to ½ in (1cm) thick. Cut into 16. Place on a baking sheet.
**3.** Bake at 425°F/220°C (Gas Mark 7) for 25 minutes. Allow to cool on a wire rack.

Each scone contains 10g CHO and 75 calories.

*Note:* This recipe freezes well.

# Prune Nut Scones

Makes 14      Total CHO — 210g      Total Cals — 1260

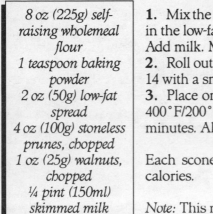

8 oz (225g) self-
raising wholemeal
flour
1 teaspoon baking
powder
2 oz (50g) low-fat
spread
4 oz (100g) stoneless
prunes, chopped
1 oz (25g) walnuts,
chopped
¼ pint (150ml)
skimmed milk

**1.** Mix the flour and baking powder. Rub in the low-fat spread. Add fruit and nuts. Add milk. Mix to a smooth dough.
**2.** Roll out to ¾ in (2cm) thick. Cut into 14 with a small cutter.
**3.** Place on a baking sheet and bake at 400°F/200°C (Gas Mark 6) for 15-20 minutes. Allow to cool on a wire rack.

Each scone contains 15g CHO and 90 calories.

*Note:* This recipe freezes well.

# Sunflower Yogurt Scones

Makes 16      Total CHO — 160g      Total Cals — 1090

2 oz (50g) low-fat
spread
8 oz (225g) self-
raising wholemeal
flour
1 oz (25g) toasted
sunflower seeds
¼ pint (150ml)
low-fat yogurt
Sea salt

**1.** Rub the fat into the flour. Add rest of ingredients. Knead to a soft dough.
**2.** Roll out to ½ in (1cm) thick. Cut into 16.
**3.** Place on a baking sheet and bake at 425°F/220°C (Gas Mark 7) for 25 minutes. Allow to cool on a wire rack.

Each scone contains 10g CHO and 70 calories.

*Note:* This recipe freezes well.

# Mushroom and Yogurt Scones

Makes 16        Total CHO — 160g        Total Cals — 960

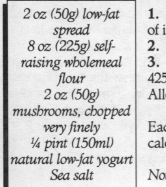

*2 oz (50g) low-fat spread*
*8 oz (225g) self-raising wholemeal flour*
*2 oz (50g) mushrooms, chopped very finely*
*¼ pint (150ml) natural low-fat yogurt*
*Sea salt*

**1.** Rub the fat into the flour. Add the rest of ingredients. Knead to a soft dough.
**2.** Roll out to ½ in (1 cm) thick. Cut into 16.
**3.** Place on a baking sheet and bake at 425°F/220°C (Gas Mark 7) for 25 minutes. Allow to cool on a wire rack.

Each scone contains 10g CHO and 60 calories.

*Note:* This recipe freezes well.

# Potato Fruit Scones        ✓

Makes 14        Total CHO — 210g        Total Cals — 1120

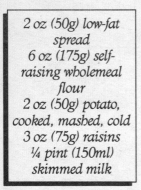

*2 oz (50g) low-fat spread*
*6 oz (175g) self-raising wholemeal flour*
*2 oz (50g) potato, cooked, mashed, cold*
*3 oz (75g) raisins*
*¼ pint (150ml) skimmed milk*

**1.** Rub the low-fat spread into the flour. Stir in the potato and raisins. Mix to a soft dough with milk.
**2.** Roll to ½ in (1cm) thick and cut into 14.
**3.** Place on a baking sheet and bake at 400°F/200°C (Gas Mark 6) for 20-25 minutes. Allow to cool on a wire rack.

Each scone contains 15g CHO and 80 calories.

*Note:* This recipe freezes well.

# Raisin and Carrot Scones ✓

Makes 18 scones    Total CHO — 180g    Total Cals — 1120

2 oz (50g) low-fat
spread
8 oz (225g) wholemeal
flour
½ teaspoon sea salt
2 teaspoons baking
powder
3 teaspoons Canderel
Spoonful or ¼
teaspoon Diamin
2 oz (50g) raisins
2 oz (50g) carrot,
grated
¼ teaspoon nutmeg
1 size 3 egg
4 tablespoons
skimmed milk

**1.** Rub the fat into the flour, salt and baking powder. Add other dry ingredients. Beat egg and milk and add this to the dry ingredients.

**2.** Roll out to ½ in (1cm) thick and cut into 18. Place on a baking sheet and bake at 400°F/200°C (Gas Mark 6) for 15 minutes. Allow to cool on a wire rack.

Each scone is 10g CHO and 65 calories.

*Note:* This recipe freezes well.

# Orange and Apricot Scone Circle

Cuts into 10     Total CHO — 200g     Total Cals — 1000

2 oz (50g) dried
apricots, chopped
Juice and rind of
1 large orange
8 oz (225g) self-
raising wholemeal
flour
1 teaspoon baking
powder
1 oz (25g) low-fat
spread
¼ pint (150ml)
skimmed milk

**1.** Soak apricots and rind in juice for 1 hour.
**2.** Mix flour and baking powder, rub in low-fat spread. Add milk and apricot mixture. Mix to a smooth dough.
**3.** Knead to a circle 1 in (2cm) thick. Mark into 10. Place on a baking tray. Bake at 350°F/180°C (Gas Mark 4) for 20-30 minutes. Allow to cool on a wire rack.

Each portion contains 20g CHO and 100 calories.

*Note:* This recipe freezes well.

# Prune Shortbread Fingers

Makes 8 fingers     Total CHO — 120g     Total Cals — 1120

5 oz (150g) 81% self-
raising flour
3 oz (75g)
polyunsaturated
margarine
2 oz (50g) stoned
prunes, very finely
chopped

**1.** Beat all ingredients together (preferably in a food processor) until they start to come together.
**2.** Press into a lightly oiled 6 in (15cm) square tin. Bake at 300°F/150°C (Gas Mark 2) for 20 minutes. Cut into fingers and allow to cool on a wire rack.

Each finger contains 15g CHO and 140 calories.

*Note:* This recipe freezes well.

# Raisin Biscuits

| Makes 10 | Total CHO — 100g | Total Cals — 1450 |

4 oz (100g) polyunsaturated margarine
2 oz (50g) fructose (fruit sugar)
1 size 3 egg
A few drops of vanilla essence
4 oz (100g) wholemeal flour
½ teaspoon bicarbonate of soda
½ teaspoon sea salt
2 oz (50g) raisins

**1.** Beat the margarine and fructose until light and fluffy. Beat in the egg and vanilla essence. Stir in the flour, soda and salt. Add the raisins.
**2.** Place teaspoons of mixture on a lightly oiled baking sheet, flatten with a damp fork. Bake at 350°F/180°C (Gas Mark 4) for 10 minutes. Allow to cool on a wire rack.

Each biscuit contains 10g CHO and 145 calories.

*Note:* This recipe freezes well.

# Coconut Crunchies ✓

Makes 30     Total CHO — 150g     Total Cals — 2200

---

*1 teaspoon
bicarbonate of soda
1 tablespoon warm
water
4 oz (100g)
polyunsaturated
margarine
1 tablespoon golden
syrup
4 oz (100g) self-
raising wholemeal
flour
4 oz (100g) oats
1 oz (25g) fructose
(fruit sugar)
4 oz (100g) desiccated
coconut*

**1.** Dissolve the soda in warm water. Leave it to stand. Melt the margarine and syrup. Mix in the remaining ingredients — mix well to ensure an even distribution of the bicarbonate of soda.

**2.** Roll the dough into small balls, flatten slightly. Place on a lightly oiled baking tray. Bake at 300°F/150°C (Gas Mark 2) for 20 minutes. Allow to cool on a wire rack.

Each biscuit contains 5g CHO and 75 calories.

*Note:* This recipe freezes well.

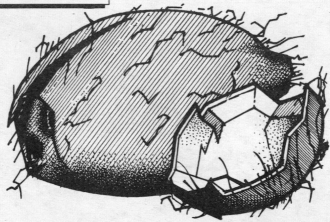

# Sesame Seed Biscuits ✓

| Makes 12 | Total CHO — 60g | Total Cals — 780 |
| --- | --- | --- |

*2 oz (50g) low-fat spread*
*3 oz (75g) self-raising wholemeal flour*
*½ oz (12g) fructose (fruit sugar)*
*2 oz (50g) sesame seeds to coat*

**1.** Rub the low-fat spread into the flour and fructose until a smooth dough forms.
**2.** Knead well, form into 12 equal sized balls. Flatten out into circles. Coat with sesame seeds. Place on a non-stick baking sheet.
**3.** Bake at 350°F/180°C (Gas Mark 4) for 10-15 minutes. (They crisp up on cooling.) Allow to cool on a wire rack.

Each biscuit contains 5g CHO and 65 calories.

*Note:* These biscuits freeze well.

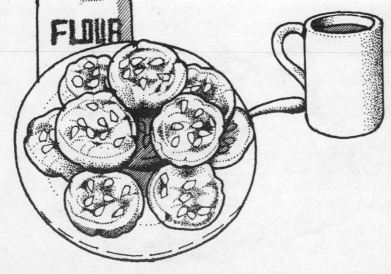

# Banana Oat Biscuits

Makes 12     Total CHO — 180g     Total Cals — 1860

4 oz (100g)
polyunsaturated
margarine
2 oz (50g) fructose
(fruit sugar)
4 oz (100g) oats
4 oz (100g) wholemeal
flour
½ teaspoon baking
powder
1 size 3 egg
2 bananas, thinly
sliced

**1.** Cream the margarine and fructose until light and fluffy. Mix in oats, flour, baking powder and egg.
**2.** Press half of the mixture into a lightly oiled 8 in (20cm) square tin. Cover with banana. Cover with the rest of the dough.
**3.** Bake at 375°F/190°C (Gas Mark 5) for 15-20 minutes. Cut into fingers and allow to cool on a wire rack.

Each biscuit contains 15g CHO and 155 calories.

*Note:* This recipe freezes well.

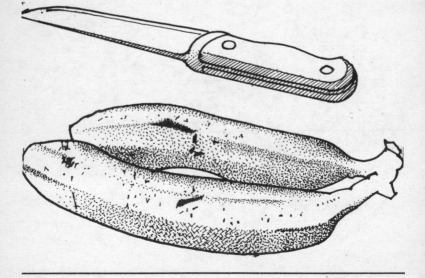

# Digestives

Makes 8 large *or* 16 small
Total CHO — 80g          Total Cals — 850

4 oz (100g) self-raising wholemeal flour
1 oz (25g) oats
2 oz (50g) low-fat spread
1 oz (25g) fructose (fruit sugar)
1 teaspoon vegetable oil

**1.** Mix all ingredients well until a soft dough forms.
**2.** Roll into a sausage shape and then slice off biscuits, making either 8 large ones or 16 small, flatten slightly. Place on a non-stick baking sheet.
**3.** Bake at 350°F/180°C (Gas Mark 4) for 15-20 minutes. Allow to cool on a wire rack.

Each biscuit contains 10g CHO and 110 calories — large; *or* 5g CHO and 55 calories — small.

*Note:* This recipe freezes well.

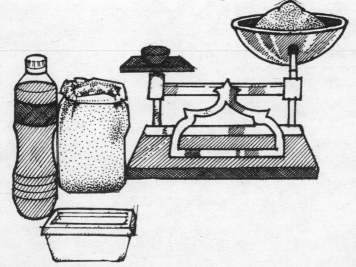

# Oatmeal Cookies          ✓

Makes 25 biscuits    Total CHO — 250g    Total Cals — 1670

*5 oz (150g) wholemeal
flour
Pinch of sea salt
Pinch of baking
powder
Pinch of baking soda
Pinch of cinnamon
Pinch of nutmeg
2 oz (50g) raisins
7 oz (200g) oatmeal
8 teaspoons* Canderel
Spoonful *or 1
teaspoon* Diamin
*2 oz (50g) low-fat
spread, melted
½ size 3 egg, beaten
1/5 pint (100ml)
skimmed milk*

**1.** Combine the dry ingredients. Beat in fat and fluids.

**2.** Shape into 25 equal size pieces and flatten slightly. Place on a lightly oiled baking tray and bake at 400°F/200°C (Gas Mark 6) for 10 minutes. Allow to cool on a wire rack.

Each biscuit contains 10g CHO and 65 calories.

*Note:* This recipe freezes well.

# 6. Soups

It is often nice to take something warm with you as part of a meal or snack. Served with a wholemeal roll these soups are substantial enough to form a good part of a meal.

## Oaty Vegetable Soup

Serves 6    Total CHO — 85g    Total Cals — 600

*1 potato, chopped*
*2 onions, chopped*
*2 carrots, chopped*
*1 small turnip,*
*chopped*
*1 leek, chopped*
*1 oz (25g)*
*polyunsaturated*
*margarine*
*2 oz (50g) rolled oats*
*1 pint (550ml) stock*
*Sea salt and freshly*
*ground black pepper*

**1.** Place all vegetables in a large pan with the margarine. Gently cook for 5 minutes.
**2.** Add remaining ingredients and simmer until the vegetables are tender (about 20-30 minutes).

Each portion contains about 15g CHO and 100 calories.

*Note:* This recipe is *not* suitable for freezing.

# Lentil and Yogurt Soup

Serves 6    Total CHO — 120g    Total Cals — 960

8 oz (225g) lentils,
soaked overnight
4 oz (100g) lean ham,
chopped
1 large carrot, peeled
and grated
1 onion, peeled and
chopped
1 pint (550ml)
chicken stock
1 teaspoon ground
coriander
2 teaspoons Worcester
sauce
Sea salt and freshly
ground black pepper
8 tablespoons natural
yogurt

**1.** Bring the lentils to the boil in fresh water. Simmer for 45 minutes.
**2.** Place the ham, carrot, onion and stock into a pan and bring to the boil. Simmer for 30 minutes.
**3.** Add the cooked lentils, coriander and Worcester sauce. Liquidize until smooth. Return to the heat and bring to the boil. Allow to cool slightly, stir in the yogurt and serve.

Each portion contains 20g CHO and 160 calories.

Note: This recipe is not suitable for freezing.

# Carrot and Potato Soup ✓

| Serves 6 | Total CHO — 60g | Total Cals — 275 |

8 oz (225g) potato, peeled and chopped
8 oz (225g) carrot, peeled and chopped
1 onion, peeled and chopped
1 stick celery, sliced
Sea salt and freshly ground black pepper
Dash of lemon juice
1 pint (550ml) stock

Bring all ingredients to the boil, simmer for 20 minutes or until the vegetables are tender. Liquidize until smooth.

Each portion contains 10g CHO and 45 calories.

Note: This recipe freezes well.

# Vegetable Mulligatawny Soup ✓

| Serves 6 | Total CHO — 150g | Total Cals — 700 |

1 oz (25g) low-fat spread
1 large onion, sliced
1 large carrot, sliced
1 large cooking apple, peeled and diced
8 oz (225g) sweet potato
8 oz (225g) potato
2 pints (1100ml) stock
2 oz (50g) sultanas
1 pinch chilli pepper
2 teaspoons curry powder

**1.** Melt the low-fat spread, sauté the onion, carrot and apple for 2-3 minutes, then add seasonings, stock, sultanas and other vegetables and bring to the boil.
**2.** Simmer for 1 hour in a covered pan, or pressure cook at 15 lb (HIGH) for 15 minutes. Allow to cool then liquidize in food processor or blender or pass through a sieve.

Each portion contains 25g CHO and 115 calories.

Note: This recipe freezes well.

# Chick Pea and Lemon Soup

Serves 4      Total CHO — 40g      Total Cals — 200

*9 oz (250g) tinned chick peas or 5 oz (150g) dried chick peas, soaked overnight*
*1 pint (550ml) stock (chicken or vegetable)*
*1 teaspoon lemon juice*
*1 large onion, chopped*
*1 tablespoon fresh parsley, chopped*

**1.** Cook the soaked dried peas in water for 30 minutes in a covered pan or pressure cook at 15 lb (HIGH) for 10 minutes and then drain *or* drain 'tinned' peas.
**2.** Cook peas, parsley, stock, lemon juice and onion in covered pan for 1 hour or pressure cook at 15 lb (HIGH) for 30 minutes. Allow to cool and purée in a blender or through a sieve. Do *not* use a processor, blending needs to be very fine.

Each portion contains 10g CHO and 50 calories.

*Note:* This recipe is *not* suitable for freezing.

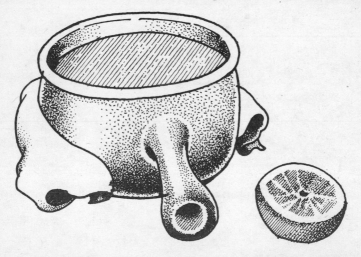

# Vegetable and Pasta Soup ✓

| Serves 4 | Total CHO — 100g | Total Cals — 500 |

3 oz (75g) tinned
kidney beans or
1½ oz (37g) dried
beans* soaked
overnight
3 oz (75g) tinned
white haricot beans or
1½ oz (37g) dried
beans soaked
overnight
½ large onion, peeled
and diced
2 large carrots, peeled
and diced
4 stalks celery, diced
4 oz (100g) potato,
peeled and diced
6 oz (175g) tomatoes
2 oz (50g) wholewheat
pasta shells/shapes/
macaroni
1¾ pints (975ml)
stock
½ teaspoon oregano
Sea salt and freshly
ground black pepper
1 oz (25g) wholemeal
flour

**1.** Cook the dried soaked beans in water with onion and half the stock for half an hour. (Otherwise drain tinned beans and add stock.) Then, for both types of beans, cook for 1 hour until beans are tender.

**2.** Cook all other vegetables in remaining stock for 20-30 minutes until tender — add pasta when water is boiling.

**3.** Combine vegetables, pasta and beans. Mix a little stock with the flour, return to the soup and thicken — simmering for 5 minutes. Adjust seasoning before serving.

Each portion contains 25g CHO and 125 calories.

Note: This recipe freezes well.

*Ensure that dried soaked red kidney beans are boiled for at least 10 minutes prior to using in any recipe.

# Orange and Carrot Soup   ✓

---

Serves 5      Total CHO — 50g      Total Cals — 240

---

1 small onion, diced
1 lb (450g) carrots
2 oranges, rind and
    juice only
1 pint (550ml) water
½ oz (12g) low-fat
    spread
Sea salt and freshly
ground black pepper

**1.** Sauté the onion, carrot and orange rind (grated) for 2-3 minutes.
**2.** Slowly add the juice, water and seasoning and bring to the boil. Boil covered for 1 hour or pressure cook 15 lb (HIGH) for 10 minutes.
**3.** Cool and purée in a blender or sieve until fine — do not use a food processor.

Each portion contains 10g CHO and 50 calories.

*Note:* This recipe freezes well.

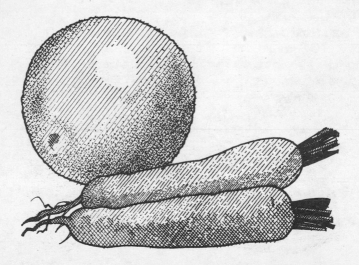

# Celery Soup

| Serves 3 | Total CHO — 30g | Total Cals — 230 |
|----------|-----------------|------------------|

*1 oz (25g) low-fat
spread
1 small onion, peeled
and chopped
1 large head of celery,
roughly chopped and
leaves
1 bayleaf
Sea salt and freshly
ground black pepper
1½ pints (825ml)
stock
4 oz (100g) sweetcorn
— frozen or tinned*

**1.** Melt fat and sauté onion and celery for 2-3 minutes, then add bayleaf, seasoning and stock.
**2.** Simmer in covered pan for 45 minutes or pressure cook on 15 lb (HIGH) for 10 minutes.
**3.** Allow to cool and remove bayleaf, add sweetcorn. Purée soup in blender, food processor or through sieve.

Each portion contains 10g CHO and 80 calories.

*Note:* This recipe freezes well.

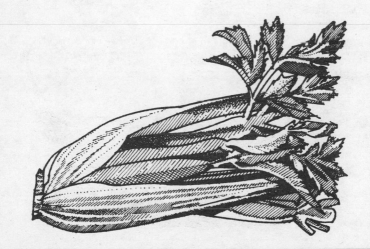

# Minestrone ✓

| Serves 8 | Total CHO — 70g | Total Cals — 440 |

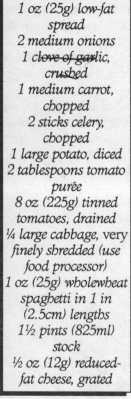

1 oz (25g) low-fat
spread
2 medium onions
1 clove of garlic,
crushed
1 medium carrot,
chopped
2 sticks celery,
chopped
1 large potato, diced
2 tablespoons tomato
purée
8 oz (225g) tinned
tomatoes, drained
¼ large cabbage, very
finely shredded (use
food processor)
1 oz (25g) wholewheat
spaghetti in 1 in
(2.5cm) lengths
1½ pints (825ml)
stock
½ oz (12g) reduced-
fat cheese, grated

**1.** Melt the low-fat spread, sauté the onions and garlic with all vegetables except the cabbage. Cook for 5 minutes. Add purée, stock, cabbage and bring to the boil.
**2.** Add spaghetti and cook covered for 25-30 minutes or pressure cook at 15 lb (HIGH) for 8 minutes. Garnish with cheese.

Each portion contains about 10g CHO and 55 calories.

*Note:* This recipe freezes well.

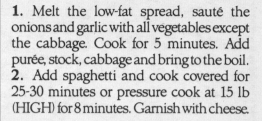

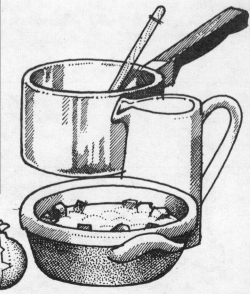

# Potato Soup  √

| Serves 4 | Total CHO — 60g | Total Cals — 250 |
|---|---|---|

½ oz (12g) low-fat spread
8 oz (225g) potatoes, diced
1 small carrot, diced
1 small onion, diced
¾ pint (425ml) stock
1 teaspoon mixed herbs
4 parsley stalks
2 tablespoons fresh chopped parsley
¼ pint (150ml) skimmed milk*
¼ pint (150ml) water*
½ oz (12g) wholemeal flour*

1. Melt the low-fat spread, and sauté the onion, carrot and potato for 2-3 minutes.
2. Add all other ingredients except flour and milk. Cook for 40-50 minutes in a covered pan or pressure cook at 15 lb (HIGH) for 10 minutes.
3. Allow to cool, remove stalks and purée in food processor, blender or through sieve. Add flour mixture and cook for 5 minutes until thickened.

Serve either hot or cold garnished with parsley.

Each portion contains 15g CHO and 65 calories.

Note: This recipe freezes well.

*Blended together.

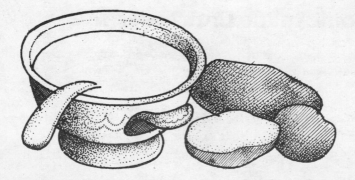

# 7. Menu Suggestions

It is important to remember that everyone has an individual diet plan which is aimed at providing an individual amount of carbohydrate and/or calories from which they must design their own meals. But it is sometimes helpful to have suggestions for possible menus. To give you some ideas of the range of foods that can be enjoyed I have produced a range of carbohydrate and calorie counted menus — which of course you can easily adapt to fit into your own particular circumstances.

Lots of our recipes freeze well (see the notes on the recipes) so if you combine foods carefully you can freeze whole lunches in advance.

## Home-made Lunches

Four home-made lunches/snacks for you to try using our recipes.

**MENU 1** — 20g CHO, under 200 Calories

|  | CHO | Cals |
|---|---|---|
| 1 Sausage Bread Roll (see page 24) | 10g | 95 |
| 1 portion Pepper Radish and Corn Salad (see page 64) | 5g | 30 |
| 1 Sesame Seed Biscuit (see page 87) | 5g | 65 |
| 1 sugar-free/low-sugar drink | neg | neg |

**MENU 2** — 30g CHO, under 250 Calories

|                                              | CHO  | Cals |
| -------------------------------------------- | ---- | ---- |
| 1 square Vegetarian Pizza (see page 26)      | 20g  | 120  |
| Celery and carrot sticks (raw)               | neg  | 20   |
| 1 Autumn Apple Slice (see page 62)           | 10g  | 105  |

*Note:* Freeze the Pizza and the Apple Slice in advance. On the day of use just add the vegetables.

**MENU 3** — 40g CHO, under 350 Calories

|                                                        | CHO  | Cals |
| ------------------------------------------------------ | ---- | ---- |
| 1 Bread Packet (see page 19)                           | 15g  | 80   |
|   with Mushroom and Herb Filling (see page 22) | neg  | 15   |
| 1 slice Stripy Chicken and Lentil Loaf (see page 47)   | 15g  | 110  |
| 1 portion Berry Curd Mousse (see page 70)              | 5g   | 60   |
| 1 Coconut Crunchy (see page 86)                        | 5g   | 75   |

**MENU 4** — 50g CHO, under 450 Calories

|                                                       | CHO  | Cals |
| ----------------------------------------------------- | ---- | ---- |
| 1 portion Oaty Vegetable Soup (see page 91)           | 15g  | 100  |
| 1 Quick Brown Roll (see page 28)                      | 15g  | 70   |
| 1 Pancake Parcel (see page 43)                        | 10g  | 60   |
|   with Kipper and Cheese Filling (see page 45) | neg  | 65   |
| 1 portion green salad                                 | neg  | 10   |
| 1 Raisin Biscuit (see page 85)                        | 10g  | 145  |

*Note:* Freeze the roll, pancake and raisin biscuit in your lunch box. On the day of use, add the soup, salad, and fill the pancake.

# Bought/home-made Lunches

Four lunches/snacks for you to try which use home-made, bought and everyday foods in healthy combinations.

**MENU 1** — 20g CHO (Snack), 125-135 Calories

| | CHO | Cals |
|---|---|---|
| 1 natural low-fat yogurt | 10g | 80 |
| 1 guava *or* 4 small dried apricots *or* | | |
| 6 oz (175g) raspberries | 10g | 45 |
| *or* (for more fibre!) Replace the fruit with | | |
| ½ oz (15g) sugar-free muesli | 10g | 55 |

**MENU 2** — 30g CHO, under 250 Calories

| | CHO | Cals |
|---|---|---|
| 1 sandwich — 2 small slices wholemeal bread | 20g | 110 |
| with 1 portion (¼ of recipe) Mackerel | | |
| Cheese Filling (see page 38) | neg | 60 |
| 1 snack bar (check values on your bar) | 10g | 75 |
| 1 sugar-free/low-sugar drink | neg | neg |

**MENU 3** — about 40g CHO, under 250 Calories

| | CHO | Cals |
|---|---|---|
| ½ wholemeal pitta | 20g | 90 |
| filled with Chinese Vegetable Filling | | |
| (½ recipe), see page 33 | neg | 5 |
| 1 peach *or* small banana *or* 15 strawberries | 10g | 40 |
| 1 'diet' yogurt | 8-13g | 85 |

**MENU 4** — 50g CHO, under 400 Calories

| | CHO | Cals |
|---|---|---|
| 1 wholemeal roll | 20g | 130 |
| filled with 1×Beef 'n' Bean Round | | |
| (see page 34) | 4g | 90 |
| 1 portion green salad | neg | 10 |
| 1 wholemeal fruited scone | 25g | 160 |

# Appendix: Food Values List

The carbohydrate and calorie contents of all the *ingredients mentioned in the book* are given so you can swap foods around and do a little experimenting of your own.

| Food | Amount | gCHO | Cals |
|------|--------|------|------|
| *All-Bran* | 1 oz (25g) | 13 | 70 |
| Apple — cooking, whole | 1 lb (450g) | 35 | 140 |
| — eating, whole | 1 | 10 | 40 |
| Apple — juice | ½ pint (275ml) | 35 | 130 |
| Apricots — dried, stoned | 1 oz (25g) | 12 | 50 |
| Aubergines, as bought | 1 lb (450g) | 11 | 50 |
| Banana, peeled | 1 medium | 10 | 40 |
| Beans — Aduki, dried, raw | 1 oz (25g) | 10 | 65 |
| — Baked | 1 oz (25g) | 3 | 20 |
| — Borlotti, tinned | 1×15 oz (425g) tin | 40 | 250 |
| — Butter, dried, raw | 1 oz (25g) | 14 | 75 |
| — Butter, tinned | 1×15 oz (425g) tin | 50 | 280 |
| — Green, fresh/frozen | 1 lb (450g) | 18 | 120 |
| — Haricot, dried | 1 oz (25g) | 13 | 80 |
| — Kidney, dried | 1 oz (25g) | 13 | 80 |
| — Kidney, tinned | 1×15 oz (425g) | 64 | 330 |
| — Soya, dried | 1 oz (25g) | 10 | 115 |
| Beansprouts, raw | 1 lb (450g) | 10 | 50 |
| Blackberries in natural juice | 1×10 oz (300g) tin | 30 | 110 |
| Bread, wholemeal | 1 oz (25g) | 12 | 60 |
| Bran — wheat | 1 oz (25g) | 5-7 | 50-60 |
| *Bran Buds* | 1 oz (25g) | 14 | 70 |

| Food | Amount | gCHO | Cals |
|---|---|---|---|
| Cabbage, raw | 1 lb (450g) | 15 | 100 |
| *Canderel Spoonful* | 1 tsp | neg | 2 |
| Carrot, raw, peeled | 1 lb (450g) | 20 | 100 |
| Celery, fresh, raw | 1 lb (450g) | 5 | 30 |
| Cheese — reduced-fat, hard | 1 oz (25g) | — | 80 |
|     — reduced-fat, soft | 1 oz (25g) | neg | 40 |
|     — reduced-fat, cottage | 1 oz (25g) | neg | 25 |
|     — cottage | 1 oz (25g) | neg | 27 |
| Chick peas, dried, raw | 1 oz (25g) | 15 | 80 |
|     — tinned | 1×15 oz (425g) tin | 60 | 280 |
| Chicken, raw, boned | 1 lb (450g) | — | 540 |
| Coconut, desiccated | 1 oz (25g) | 1-2 | 170 |
| Courgettes, raw, whole | 1 lb (450g) | 15 | 100 |
| Crab, tinned, drained | 1 oz (25g) | — | 25 |
| Cucumber, raw, as bought | 1 lb (450g) | 8 | 45 |
| Currants, dried | 1 oz (25g) | 18 | 70 |
| Dates, dried, stoned | 1 oz (25g) | 18 | 70 |
| Eggs, raw | 1×size 3 | — | 75 |
| Flour — wholemeal, plain | 1 oz (25g) | 18 | 90 |
|     — wholemeal, SR | 1 oz (25g) | 18 | 90 |
|     — 81% plain | 1 oz (25g) | 19 | 92 |
|     — 81% SR | 1 oz (25g) | 19 | 92 |
| Fructose | 1 oz (25g) | 30* | 115 |
| Gelatine | 1 sachet | — | 35 |
| Guavas, in natural juice | 1×10 oz (285g) tin | 30 | 140 |
| Ham, lean, boiled | 1 oz (25g) | — | 35 |
| Hazelnuts, shelled | 1 oz (25g) | 2 | 110 |
| Honey, clear | 1 oz (25g) | 20 | 80 |
| Kipper, fillet, raw | 1 oz (25g) | — | 60 |
| Leek, raw, as bought | 1 lb (450g) | 30 | 140 |

*Note: Usually ignored if less than 1 oz (25g) taken in one day.

| Food | Amount | gCHO | Cals |
|------|--------|------|------|
| Lentils (all varieties), raw | 1 oz (25g) | 15 | 85 |
| Low-fat spread | 1 oz (25g) | — | 105 |
| Mackerel — tinned in tomato sauce | 1 oz (25g) | — | 60 |
| Margarine — polyunsaturated | 1 oz (25g) | — | 210 |
| Melon, whole, raw | 1 lb (450g) | 13 | 60 |
| Milk, skimmed, fresh | 1 pint | 30 | 190 |
| Minced beef, lean | 1 lb (450g) | —. | 820 |
| Muesli — sugar free | 1 oz (25g) | 18 | 100 |
| Mushrooms, whole, raw | 1 lb (450g) | — | 70 |
| Oats/Oatmeal, raw | 1 oz (25g) | 20 | 110 |
| Oil | 1 fl oz | — | 255 |
| Onion, raw, as bought | 1 lb (450g) | 25 | 100 |
| Orange juice, unsweetened | ¼ pint (150ml) | 15 | 60 |
| Parsnip, raw, as bought | 1 lb (450g) | 40 | 160 |
| Pasta — wholegrain, raw, dry | 1 oz (25g) | 19 | 95 |
| Peaches, in natural juice | 1×14 oz (411g) tin | 45 | 180 |
| Peanuts, shelled | 1 oz (25g) | 2 | 160 |
| Peanut butter, smooth | 1 oz (25g) | 5 | 160 |
| Pepper, green or red, raw | 1 lb (450g) | 8 | 60 |
| Pineapple, in natural juice | 1×15 oz (425g) tin | 55 | 240 |
| Potato, raw, as bought | 1 lb (450g) | 80 | 340 |
| Prunes — stoned, dried, whole | 1 oz (25g) | 10 | 40 |
| Quark cheese | 1 oz (25g) | 1½ | 25 |
| Radishes, raw, as bought | 1 oz (25g) | neg | 5 |
| Raisins, dried | 1 oz (25g) | 18 | 70 |
| Salad cream — low calorie | 1 tblsp | 3 | 15 |
| Sardines in tomato sauce | 1×120g tin | 1 | 210 |
| Sausagemeat — pork, good quality | 1 lb (450g) | 45 | 1575 |
| Semolina | 1 oz (25g) | 18 | 100 |
| Sesame seeds | 1 oz (25g) | 5 | 160 |

| Food | Amount | gCHO | Cals |
|------|--------|------|------|
| Spinach, boiled and drained or frozen, thawed and drained | 1 lb (450g) | 6 | 140 |
| Spring onions, raw | 1 lb (450g) | 23 | 105 |
| Strawberries, fresh | 1 lb (450g) | 27 | 110 |
| Sultanas, dried | 1 oz (25g) | 18 | 70 |
| Sunflower seeds | 1 oz (25g) | 5 | 160 |
| Sweetcorn, tinned, kernels | 1×11 oz (133g) tin | 55 | 250 |
| Sweet potato, raw, as bought | 1 lb (450g) | 80 | 350 |
| Syrup, golden | 1 oz (25g) | 22 | 85 |
| Tomatoes — canned | 1×14 oz (405g) tin | 10 | 50 |
| — fresh | 1 lb (450g) | 10 | 60 |
| Tomato purée | 1 oz (25g) | 4 | 20 |
| Tuna, in brine | 1×7 oz (120g) tin | — | 220 |
| Turnip, raw, as bought | 1 lb (450g) | 15 | 90 |
| Vegetable fat, white | 1 oz (25g) | — | 255 |
| Walnuts, shelled | 1 oz (25g) | 1½ | 150 |
| Yeast, dried | 1 sachet | neg | neg |
| Yogurt, low-fat natural | 1×5 oz (150g) | 10 | 80 |

# Recommended Reading

These books contain lots of helpful information and many recipes which you can use in your packed lunches and snacks.

*Countdown*
(Published by British Diabetic Association)
A guide to carbohydrate and calorie content of manufactured foods.

*Better Cookery for Diabetics*
(Published by British Diabetic Association)
A recipe book by Jill Metcalfe.

*Cooking the New Diabetic Way*
(Published by British Diabetic Association)
A recipe book by Jill Metcalfe.

*Simple Diabetic Cookery*
(Published by British Diabetic Association)
A recipe leaflet.

*Simple Home Baking*
(Published by British Diabetic Association)
A recipe leaflet.

*The Vegetarian on a Diet*
(Published by Thorsons Publishing Group, 1984)
A recipe book for vegetarians by Margaret Cousins and Jill Metcalfe.

# Further Information

## BRITISH DIABETIC ASSOCIATION

Diabetes affects just over two per cent of the population of the UK. Although it cannot be cured or prevented, it can be controlled by proper treatment.

The British Diabetic Association (BDA) was formed in 1934 to help all diabetics, to overcome prejudice and ignorance about diabetes, and to raise money for research towards a cure. The Association is currently budgeting £1m each year to this end, and is the largest single contributor to diabetic research in the U.K.

The Association is an independent organization with over 100,000 members and 300 local branches. It provides a welfare and advisory service for diabetics and their families. It also liaises closely with those who work in the field of diabetes.

Educational and activity holidays are organized for diabetics of all ages plus parent/child and parent/teenager weekends.

Members receive the BDA's bi-monthly magazine *Balance* which keeps readers up to date with news of the latest research and all aspects of diabetes.

All diabetics have to follow a lifelong diet and *Balance* publishes recipes and dietary information to help bring interest and variety in eating.

To become a member, fill in the application form and send it with your subscription to:

British Diabetic Association,
10 Queen Anne Street,
London W1M 0BD.
Tel: 01-323 1531

# Enrolment Form

British Diabetic Association
10 Queen Anne Street
London W1M 0BD

## MEMBERSHIP SUBSCRIPTIONS

Life membership — Single payment of £105 or £15 a year for 7 years under covenant

Annual membership — £5.00 a year

Pensioner Membership — £1.00 a year

Reduced Rate Membership — widowed, disabled, on government grant, etc. — £1.00 a year

Overseas annual membership — £10.00 a year

Overseas life membership — Single payment of £150.00

---

Please enrol me as a:

☐ Life member: £105 £15 a year for 7 years under covenant

☐ Annual member: £5.00

☐ Pensioner member: £1.00

☐ Overseas annual member: £10.00

☐ Overseas Life member: £150.00

☐ Are you joining on behalf of a child? (Children in the UK under the age of 16 can join free for one year if they wish)

I enclose Remittance/Banker's Order/Covenant for £ ...............................
(Please delete whichever does not apply)

Date ...................................... Signature ..........................

Full name: Mr/Mrs/Miss ...................................................
(Block Capitals please)

Address ...............................................................

................................................................

Date of Birth ..................................... Occupation ....................
(This information will be treated as strictly confidential)

## COVENANT

I/we,...............................................................................(full name), of
...........................................................................................(address)
covenant with the British Diabetic Association that for four ☐ or
seven years ☐ from the present date or during my lifetime (whichever
period shall the shorter) I/we will pay to the Association on the
...........................................................................................(this date
should be the same as, or later than, the date of the signature) in every
year such a sum as, after deduction of income tax for the time being
in force, amounts to £.............................................................
(insert actual amount you wish to pay).
(Indicate by tick in box).

Signed, sealed and delivered by me/us this..........day of...........19......
Signature..........................................................................
Signature of witness............................................................
Address of witness..............................................................

---

## BANKER'S ORDER

To.................................Bank.............................Branch,
...........................................................................................(address)
Date.................................................Please pay to the National
Westminster Bank Ltd, 154 Harley Street, London W1 (60 10 02) now
and on...................................(date) each year for four years ☐,
seven years ☐ or until further notice ☐ the sum of...........................
pounds for the credit of the British Diabetic Association
(A/c No. 12773085)                 (Indicate by tick in box)

Signed.............................................................................

Name................................................................................
(Block Capitals Please)

Address............................................................................
..........................................A/c No............................................

*Please return the completed Covenant/Banker's Order to:*
**BRITISH DIABETIC ASSOCIATION**
**10 Queen Anne Street, London W1M 0BD. Tel: 01-323 1531.**

# Index